Social Policy and Health Care FAIRFIELD GENERAL HOSPITAL
LIBRARY

For Churchill Livingstone:

Commissioning Editor: Ellen Green
Project Manager: Valerie Burgess; Ewan Halley
Project Development Editor: Mairi McCubbin
Design direction: Judith Wright

Social Policy and Health Care

Edited by

Kevin Gormley RGN RMN ONC RCNT RNT BA MSc
Nurse Lecturer, School of Nursing and Midwifery, Queen's University of Belfast, Belfast

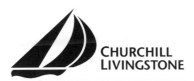

CHURCHILL
LIVINGSTONE

EDINBURGH LONDON NEW YORK PHILADELPHIA SYDNEY TORONTO 1999

CHURCHILL LIVINGSTONE
An imprint of Harcourt Brace and Company Limited

© Harcourt Brace and Company Limited 1999

⟁ is a registered trade mark of Harcourt Brace and
Company Limited

First edition 1999

ISBN 0 443 057478

British Library of Cataloguing in Publication Data
A catalogue record for this book is available from the British
Library.

Library of Congress Cataloging in Publication Data
A catalogue record for this book is available from the
Library of Congress

Medical knowledge is constantly changing. As new
information becomes available, changes in treatment,
procedures, equipment and the use of drugs become
necessary. The editor, the contributors and the publishers
have, as far as it is possible, taken care to ensure that the
information given in this text is accurate and up to date.
However, readers are strongly advised to confirm that the
information, especially with regard to drug usage, complies
with latest legislation and standards of practice.

The
publisher's
policy is to use
**paper manufactured
from sustainable forests**

Printed in China
EPC/01

Contents

Contributors

Owen Barr BSc(Hons) PGDipCan RGN RNMH CNMH ADDIPEd
Lecturer in Nursing, University of Ulster, Coleraine
10 Learning disabilities and mental health
11 Children

Kevin Gormley RGN RMN ONC RCNT RNT BA MSc
Nurse Lecturer, The Queen's University of Belfast, Belfast
1 Introduction
2 The development of health and social care services
3 The nurse and the welfare state
7 Reorganised health care
9 Disability
13 Future trends

Simon Smith MPhil MSc DipNurs (Lond) ADDipEdStudies RGN
Nurse Lecturer, Queen's University of Belfast, Belfast
12 International health care provision

Fred Sutton BSc MSc
Research Fellow, University of Warwick, Coventry
1 Introduction
4 The process of policy implementation
8 The mixed economy of healthcare
13 Future trends

Julie S. Taylor RGN BSc(Hons) MSc RNT
Researcher/Lecturer, University of Dundee, Dundee
11 Children,
13 Future trends

Siân P. Thomas MA GradIPD
Research and Information Officer, Royal College of Nursing, Edinburgh
5 Social issues and health
6 Gender issues

Preface

The education process for health care students generally aims to provide them with competencies that will assist them in carrying out their role. Sometimes, however, this process fails, especially in assisting students to develop their own attitudes towards political matters that affect the distribution of services to meet the needs of the patient. This is where a social policy module can prove helpful, particularly as managerial roles within the health services require individuals to have a clear understanding of the nature of health care provision.

Until recently, social policy issues that affected health care were either ignored or taught *ad hoc*, if there was a teacher on site who had a particular interest in the subject. Now, social policy modules have been introduced into many undergraduate programmes for health care professionals. They aim to give health care professionals a political awareness that did not previously exist, to enable them to play a more decisive and interactive role in the process of policy development and implementation, and to stimulate a wider academic interest in the subject, particularly amongst those involved in teaching it.

The dearth of textbooks providing students with a good foundation of information, encouraging further reading and knowledge gain, has encouraged the authors to write this book. Most are experienced lecturers with a specific interest in health care issues affecting current social policies and have focused specifically on the needs of health care undergraduate students. In planning

the content, the authors have recognised that the potential readership is not intending to pursue a career in social policy. The content has therefore been kept within the pre-existing maps of their needs, focussing mainly on the patient. The topics reveal the dilemmas that governments encounter in attempting to provide services that are universal, equitable and justly distributed. The book also concentrates on specific government policies and on provision for specific client groups that students will encounter during their day-to-day working experience.

Social Policy and Health Care provides the reader with an insight into the processes that led to the emergence of universal health care, offers an authoritative review and critique of current social policy and its effects on health care provision, and forecasts future directions. The most important changes that have emerged are described in a clear, jargon-free style, and the individuals who influenced these changes are looked at.

Most academic subjects need to be confrontational, argumentative and interactive, and this is especially the case with social policy. The interactive text aims to provoke or stimulate the reader to question and form a personal view of policy decisions. The design and structure of the text is intentionally reader-friendly in the sequencing of chapters, inclusion of study activities and the provision of an extensive reference section.

The book should be a valuable resource for students and lecturers involved in social policy modules. It should also be a useful foundation text for other health care programmes that address health care policy issues. Health care professionals who are involved in the development of health care policy may also benefit from reading and working through this text.

Belfast, 1998   Kevin Gormley

1 Introduction

Fred Sutton   Kevin Gormley

At the end of the chapter the student will be able to:

- **understand the purpose of social policy**
- **understand the aims and constraints on social policy**
- **appreciate the importance of social policy as a curricular subject**

Introduction

It could be argued that the changes currently taking place in terms of health economics, mixed markets and quality of care packages will be more dramatic than the combined changes of the last half century. The development of health care reforms and the emergence of new services aim to provide better health care, greater efficiency, accountability and choice, and an increase in consumer orientation. If health care professionals are to keep pace and react appropriately to these changes they must appreciate the dynamics that underpin policies. They must also be open-minded enough to to accept the diversity of need among patients that is now apparent within health and social care services. This chapter will introduce the concepts of social policy and the aims behind the policies, and why these will differ when seen from differing political viewpoints. It will examine constraints on social policy and how policies are aimed at certain groups and their problems (Department of Health 1991, Klein 1983, McCarthy 1990).

Modern curicula used as a basis for teaching

and preparing health care professionals focus on introducing to the student a sense of self-enquiry and flexibility, as well as imparting a sound understanding of the practice of health care from a basis of research and societal appreciation. It is within this framework that the importance of social policy as a curricular subject is best understood. Social policy is a broad subject; it is therefore vital that the content of a social policy unit in the preregistration curriculum is placed within pre-existing maps of knowledge. In health care, the most appropriate focus is patients and the divergent needs and backgrounds from which they come.

WHAT IS SOCIAL POLICY?

The study of social policy is the study of social welfare and of the health and social services. Social policy is the means of organising the nation's resources for the 'perceived benefit' of society. The perception of what most benefits society is dependent on who is in charge of policy and on what they consider to be beneficial. The main areas of social policy studies are policy and administrative practices in health, social security, education, employment services, community care and housing management; the circumstances in which people's welfare is likely to be impaired, including disability, unemployment, mental illness, learning disability and old age; social problems like crime; issues relating to social disadvantage, including race, gender and poverty; and the range of collective social responses to these circumstances (Spicker 1995, p. 4). The core elements of policy are its origins, its goals, the process of implementation and the results. Social policy does not study a particular subject, but looks at how it is provided and achieved (for example social policy is not concerned with physical health, but with policies to promote health and with the provision of health care services).

The study of social policy as an academic discipline has its roots in the early years of the 20th century, at a time when fundamental moral and social questions were being debated with a renewed sense of vigour and purpose. Titmuss (1963) describes how the focus of enquiry moved from 'Who are the poor and neglected in society?' to 'Why are they poor and what are the resultant effects of poverty in terms of health and well-being?'. As an area of academic study social policy is underpinned by many other subjects including sociology, politics and philosophy, and from these creates its own discrete body of knowledge. Using these subjects, social policy theorists question the nature and philosophy of those government interventions designed to protect and provide a reasonable lifestyle for all of the country's citizens.

Social problems

Social policy is sometimes represented as responses to social problems. Social problems do indeed present issues which require some response. However, it is not always the case that everyone agrees on what constitutes a problem. The definition of a problem varies in different places, and the nature of that problem needs to be understood in order for a response to be made. People may understand issues differently; for example they may differ in what they believe are the causes of crime. Some may say that crime is caused by a failure to instil moral fibre in young people, some may believe that underlying poverty is the problem, whereas others may say that it is due to leniency in law and order. Depending on the viewpoint of policy makers as to what they believe the causes of crime to be, then the policies they implement to 'solve' the problem will differ.

The nature of social problems

Social problems are problems that may not just affect individuals but which may also affect society as a whole. They tend to arise from individual human needs. Some needs are obvious, such as the need for food and clothing, whereas others are more conceptual, such as the need for status in society. These common human needs are met largely by personal and family action: individuals work for their living, find accommodation, establish friendships and obtain care, security and a sense of purpose within family and social groups. But when these needs are not met, this gives rise to problems. The basic need to subsist leads to the social problem of poverty whenever families and individuals are unable to meet that need themselves. Likewise, the common need for shelter, if unmet, is the basis of the housing problem (Brown 1994).

Activity

Discuss with your study group the value of studying social policy when preparing to become a health care professional.

Welfare

Social policy is concerned with welfare. Welfare can mean well-being and social policy can be represented as being concerned with well-being in general, although it would be more accurate to say that social policy is concerned with people who lack well-being, people with particular kinds of problems or needs, and the services which provide for them (Box 1.1). The boundaries are indistinct because often people's needs have to be understood in terms of the facilities available to others; our idea of good housing, adequate income or good health affects our view of what people need or what we consider constitutes a problem. What we may agree as being poor housing in our society will not necessarily be the same as in other societies.

Individualism and collectivism

There is a debate over whether welfare should

> **Box 1.1 Fundamental issues of social policy**
>
> - Health and disease
> - Social care
> - Education
> - Housing
> - Poverty
> - Employment
> - Crime and justice

---

be taken at an individual or a collective level. The welfare of individuals is increased by examining the circumstances of each individual, to see whether or not that person can be said to be better or worse off. One view of social welfare is that it is made up of the sum of the people's welfare; in the case of public goods like parks or roads collective action can yield more benefit for each person than the cost to each individual user. But there is also the view that societies have interests and welfare which are distinct from that of any individual member.

The welfare of society If welfare is interpreted on a collective level then there are different criteria by which the welfare needs of a society ought to be judged. Societies can be said to have needs in the sense that there are things which are necessary for a society to survive. Societies have to maintain order to deal with change and to reproduce themselves for the future. Spending on education may be irrelevant to someone who has no children, but for the welfare of society as a whole to increase it needs an educated labour force. Societies need people to work, so spending on education, social security and health care can all be seen as helping to maintain the workforce.

Activities

- List five areas where you believe that the state should intervene to ensure a satisfactory lifestyle for its citizens.
- Consider whether there is an alternative to state intervention in these areas.
- Select one area of public service and discuss with your friends what would happen if this service was abruptly discontinued.

DECISION AND ACTION IN SOCIAL POLICY

The study of policy examines both formal decisions and actions. A decision by itself is not an action; it is the result of that decision that is the action. What happens in practice may be different from what was intended by decision makers, and indeed the implementation of a policy may have the opposite effect to the one intended, so that the implementation of a policy can be just as important as how that policy was decided on in the first place.

Policy implementation may involve a number of decisions as opposed to one main decision or it may be the selection of one possibility from a number of others. A policy may be chosen not for its effectiveness at alleviating a particular problem but for its cost effectiveness. Policy tends to be defined in terms of a number of decisions which, taken together, comprise an understanding of what the policy is. Along with this, policies change over time for various reasons. Yesterday's policy goals may not be the same as today's, and policy can change as perceived attitudes change or because the previous goals have been met. After a mass vaccination programme has been carried out and the number of cases of the disease has reduced to a tiny amount then there is no need to continue the policy on such a massive scale. Along with policy implementation there is policy stagnation; this is where political activity is concerned with maintaining the status quo, and resisting challenges to upset the apple cart by reallocating resources to a policy that may be unpopular.

Activities

- Consider one area of the public service that you feel is under-resourced and jot down some ideas as to how you would channel extra resources to meet this need.
- Now write down what the net effect of this would be.
- Organise a seminar with your class to discuss the allocation of resources for public services.

DIRECTION OF SOCIAL POLICY

Since social policy is concerned with helping people, how are policies devised and directed at those individuals or groups perceived to be in need of assistance? It would be almost impossible to assess the needs of every single individual in the country, and so it is necessary to assign people to certain groups. Although the idea that people are individuals is widely held, we do not live in a social vacuum. We grow up in families and the way in which we develop and live is conditioned by others, be they members of the family, friends, work colleagues, etc. In this way individuals will share some of the same characteristics, whilst still retaining their identity as individuals.

People can be classified into groups in a variety of ways. The groups may be individuals who share certain characteristics, although this is not always the case. Or they could be groups of individuals seen as having similar social contacts or networks, or as occupying similar positions in society. The first refers to how people live (for example family, workplace) and explains the context in which social policies take effect. The second is concerned with the way people's situation relates to others (for example class, race and gender). It identifies the cause of people's circumstances and the constraints placed on them.

How people live

Family

The family is the basis for a great part of social interaction. This generalisation disguises a number of different functions which, conventionally, are packaged together. The idea of the family is also used to refer to many other kinds of households, where people who are not related by birth or marriage live together. The household is also an important unit, since most people live with other people, sharing or dividing up income and expenses in some way.

The term 'family' covers a whole range of groups but when used in policy it generally refers to a subset, specifically people with children.

Where there are formal family policies they tend to be policies specifically geared to families with children. The relationship between adult members of a family, like the relationship between adult children and their ageing parents, can be crucially important for policy. The provision of domiciliary support by the state is generally built around the pattern of care which a relative delivers, and recognises that that care is often greater than anything the public services can deliver. However, policy also makes assumptions that may not hold in practice. For example the 1988 Social Security Act removed the entitlement of benefit to 16–18-year-olds. This, along with the reduction of benefits to young people under the age of 25, assumes that the family will still shoulder some financial responsibility for the young person. Whether or not this happens in practice is another question.

Activity

Discuss with your friends whether social policies tend to discriminate against specific groups in society, for example young people or ethnic minorities.

Community

The term 'community' can be a vague topic, and may mean different things to different people (Box 1.2). Community can be regarded as the area in which people live, i.e. the local neighbourhood. This definition of community can be more applicable to some areas than others, depending on the degree of social interactions amongst the neighbourhood. Another way of looking at community is to define it in terms of interactions between people, even though there may not be a common geographical boundary. This would cover communities, for example, which are defined by their religious convictions. Other communities can have what may seem on the surface to be little linkage, such as the business community, which refers to a large

Box 1.2 Community

- A geographical area in which people live
- A group of people from similar ethnic background or religious belief
- A business community
- A degree of social interaction creating a community spirit

number of diverse organisations over a vast geographical spread (Spicker 1995).

Workplace

The workplace is an important place for social interaction and for the definition of work status and therefore of status and power in society. In much of Europe the workplace has been the central location from which organised social action has been developed. In a number of other countries the trade unions have become responsible for the administration of benefits and services, such as unemployment benefits in Denmark, or the health services in Israel (Spicker 1995, p. 24).

However, the importance of the workplace in social policy has diminished in recent years for a number of reasons. Firstly the state has been increasingly seen as the main route through which welfare can be provided. Where the state has failed to provide, responsibility has been undertaken primarily by women and the family. Along with this, the rise in global unemployment has removed large numbers of people from the workplace. There has also been a shift in social policy from the conditions of people in work to those that are unemployed, although even this emphasis has reduced over the last decade or more.

Activities

- Write brief notes as to what is meant by the term community.
- Organise a debate in your class to discuss what is meant by the term community.

Inequality

The problem of inequality has been one of the main issues to which social policy has been addressed in the past. Inequality refers not to the fact that people are different but that people are advantaged or disadvantaged in social terms.

This kind of advantage and disadvantage leads to differentials in access to opportunities and rewards in society.

One of the areas in which inequality exists is in resources such as income and wealth. The possession of resources is often a key access to the structure of social advantage, conversely lack of resources can imply cumulative disadvantages in material circumstances, lifestyle and opportunities. Those who possess resources are able to access alternatives to the standard services. They can enter into the private market for health care or education, for example. Those who lack resources are denied this access and the ability to extricate themselves from their position. In terms of communities, an area which lacks resources becomes less attractive to those with extra resources, and so they tend to move out of the area. This can produce a knock-on effect, with the area having even less resources so that it becomes even less attractive. In the workplace trade unions were organised to fight against inequalities, whether between employers and employees or between workers in different, or similar, industries.

Persistent inequalities

As cyclical recessions continue to recur, more people generally suffer from unemployment and ensuing poverty. The decline of regionally-based industries can have profound knock-on effects where these industries have not been replaced. Whilst manufacturing has been declining there has been an increase in the service sector. Unfortunately, these growing sectors are not always in the same locations as the declining sectors so that the relatively disadvantaged groups suffer even more. Thus certain areas will suffer disproportionately high levels of unemployment and poverty, and their frustration turns increasingly to protest. This situation demands action of a positive nature but usually provokes a repressive response.

One of the problems with inequalities is that if they continue then they can have a cumulative effect, with certain groups being continuously denied the opportunities open to others. Without these opportunities they are denied access to the standard of living enjoyed by those that are more 'equal'. The existence of inequality should not be viewed on an individual basis. That is, the status of one form of inequality cannot be assessed without comparison to another. For example the position of women cannot be understood without reference to the position of men. People are poor not simply because they do not have enough but because others have the things that they do not. The study of social policy seeks to define the nature of these relationships, along with defining measures to reduce the inequalities.

Gender Although there is a biological difference between the sexes, the social construction of gender bears little relationship to such differences. The understanding of gender divisions has become increasingly important for the analysis of social policy since a number of the traditional concerns of social welfare like poverty, health and old age have important gender-related dimensions. There has been longstanding evidence that women earn less than men for performing the same jobs. There has also been concern that the House of Commons, which is supposed to represent the people, is unrepresentative since the majority of MPs are male.

Despite the application of social policy over the years, inequalities still exist in a number of areas. With respect to gender, there are still differentials between the situation of men and women. Although the Equal Pay Act and the Sex Discrimination Act became the law in the 1970s, and the Equal Opportunities Commission was established to work towards the elimination of sex discrimination, such inequalities persist. These inequalities are prominent in the areas of employment and pay, although they also exist in other areas. In some instances this discrimination had been challenged in European courts, most notably the case of payment of social security benefits to women.

Pay between the sexes is still unevenly distributed, along with their respective job status. In recent years the traditional role of men and women in the economy has changed to some degree. The decline of male full-time employment has been accompanied by the increase of part-time work, which has generally been at a lower wage. The increase of part-time work has generally been in the service sector, while the decline in full-time employment has been in the manufacturing sector. This increase in part-time work has generally been taken up by women. There are several reasons for this, one being that there has been a regional disparity in the growth of the service sector, which has expanded in different areas to those that suffered a decline in manufacturing. Also men traditionally have been employed in full-time work and may not have adapted to the change in the labour market.

Race Race, like gender, is a socially constructed concept but, unlike gender, the term covers a wide range of different types of characteristics and it is used variously to indicate physical, cultural and/or historical differences. Different racial groups are subject to important disadvantages in society and, like women, they too have the problem of not being represented in the House of Commons.

Race Relations Acts were passed in 1968 and 1976. These were intended to strengthen the laws against discrimination on the grounds of race, making it illegal to discriminate in housing, employment and social services, etc. The Commission for Racial Equality has a duty to work towards the elimination of discrimination and the promotion of equality of opportunity and good race relations. Despite these policies there are still inequalities suffered by ethnic minorities in the UK. The implementation of social policy has failed to reduce the inequality that results from discrimination. Britain has substantial ethnic minorities which are concentrated unevenly in certain cities and areas. As a result of cumulative racial prejudice and discrimination, racial minorities are disadvantaged in terms of income levels, housing standards, employment opportunities and educational facilities (Clarke et al 1994).

The statutory response to these problems was first to control immigration, in an attempt to contain the size of the group, and then to outlaw discrimination. Although local authorities now have various powers, the extent to which they pursue positive discrimination is limited. There has been a reluctance on the part of local authorities to appear to be favouring racial minorities in the provision of housing or education services for fear of arousing a politically threatening backlash. As a result the disadvantaged position of ethnic minorities has not been much alleviated and racial discontent and tension have increased despite the Race Relations legislation.

Activities

- List five areas of society where you believe inequalities exist.
- Select any two and discuss with your teacher and colleagues in a group the reasons why these inequalities are present.

Universality and selectivity

Policy can largely be divided into two types: a universal policy or a selective policy. A universal social policy is one which aims to provide services to everyone, or at least everyone within a broadly-defined category, such as all old people or all children. A selective policy is one which focuses resources just on those people in need.

The arguments for and against universality and selectivity concern the focus of policy. Universality is seen as a way of getting resources to everyone in need (for example Child Benefit). The main problem with this approach is that resources are wasted on those who are not in need. The argument for selective policies is that if benefits were targeted then not only would less money be spent, but it would be spent to greater effect.

Identifying those in need One problem with targeting individuals is that first they need to be identified, this leads to the problem of how they are identified. If the process is self-selection, then the people in that situation have to know that they are eligible for help and how to go about applying for any benefits.

Defining limits Along with this there is a

problem of defining limits. If you fall below a certain level then you become applicable for certain benefits, but if you are just above the limit then you are not eligible and as a result may end up worse off than those who are just below the limit (Spicker 1995).

Choice

People who receive benefits have their behaviour conditioned and determined by the services available. It is usually their decision to claim, and the choices that are made by recipients are an important constituent part of demand. Choice is traditionally the mechanism through which an individual can maximise their welfare. In the operation of social services the opportunity to exercise choice has often been limited.

The market place Concerns about choices have mainly been expressed through arguments for considering the delivery of welfare in terms of a market, in which the recipients of welfare services are consumers. The central principle is that the decisions are made by the person who is likely to receive the services, rather than by someone else on their behalf.

In the operation of an economic market consumers have the opportunity to use resources to purchase goods and services. The priorities which are determined, and any resulting decisions about price and supply, arise from the interaction of many people rather than from the policy of some central authority. When people are short of food or clothing few people would argue for distribution by the state; the argument is much more commonly made that people need to have the money to pay for such items themselves. The idea that the poor might be subject to a regime in which they are unable to choose what they eat or what they wear is not a popular one. Arguments for social security or income maintenance are generally arguments to give people the money to choose, rather than deciding what they need. So although income support levels are set at a rate that the government determines as the minimum needed to subsist, recipients are still left with the choice of what they spend their money on.

Limits on choice By contrast, arguments are commonly made in discussions of housing, education or health which point to the inefficiencies and constraints on choice which arise in the private sector. The problem is not simply that people have unequal resources, which would be an argument for redistribution of income, but that the process of exercising choices leads to inequalities or inappropriate decisions. Part of that is attributable to the problems of exercising choice meaningfully. People who are desperate are not in a strong bargaining position. In health care there is the problem of knowing and understanding what is being purchased. In housing and education the effect of choice is to produce a stratified system with profound social consequences.

The recipients of welfare services tend to be disadvantaged, and they have fewer options from which choices can be made. In these circumstances the opportunity to exercise choice may simply aggravate existing disadvantages. In education parents who can afford to move into the catchment areas of the better schools are able to buy a considerable social advantage for their children. In housing social housing is nominally let according to some system of priorities in allocation, usually on the basis of need. But people who are offered social housing are usually given only a very limited choice – they might be allowed two or three chances and even then their choices are likely to be limited because they do not know what their next option will be like and they are often reluctant to accept social housing in poor areas. But some people are more able to exercise choice than others. A lot depends on whether people are able to hold on a little longer. The result is that people who are least able to exercise choice have to take what others are able to refuse, and so people who are desperate and most in need are likely to receive the worst housing.

The problem with limiting choice is that it does not necessarily guarantee that disadvantages will be redressed. The real aim is not to obstruct choices and opportunities, but to ensure that those who are poorest and most disadvantaged will be able to exercise such opportunities.

Efficiency

A policy is only effective if it succeeds in achieving what it was intended to achieve. Efficiency is not necessarily the same as effectiveness. A policy is effective when it achieves its aims to the maximum degree, and it is efficient when it does so at the minimum cost. Agencies are often able to achieve their goals, for example medical treatment or domestic support for many people. Reaching other people, however, can be more expensive, for example because their needs are greater or because they are more difficult to locate. In other words, as the service increases its caseload, the cost of each additional person helped is likely to be higher, and so its average costs are also likely to increase. The point of maximum efficiency is passed when the costs of helping the next person is greater than the cost of helping the previous one. Almost invariably this will happen before the agency has covered everyone in need, and so a concern with efficiency can reduce the effectiveness of the service.

Public services cannot usually maintain their efficiency by refusing to help people at all, although it does happen to some extent. There may be a point at which the costs of providing services are considered too great, for example some hospitals may suspend treatment to non-urgent cases when they are nearing the end of their budget: more commonly, services avoid taking on liabilities by trying to pass on expensive or difficult cases to other agencies. Continuing care for elderly people is particularly expensive because it incorporates both residential care with extended coverage. For any agency which is not specifically geared to providing such care this is an inefficient option because it greatly increases the cost of care for each patient. The only agency which would not consider it inefficient would be one specifically dedicated to the provision of such care. Thus the effect of concentrating on efficiency as a criterion is to favour the setting up of smaller agencies which are functionally differentiated. It is debatable, however, whether this is socially efficient in the sense of reducing costs across the whole of welfare provision, for cost-effective small agencies lose the economies of scale which larger agencies can achieve (for example through the use of pooled laundry services or catering). In the context of social policy an emphasis on efficiency can be misleading. Cost effectiveness is far more relevant and appropriate to the work of social services.

Conclusion

The promotion of good health and the prevention of disease requires the creation of a social and economic environment within which people can live and be healthier. Halfdan Mahler, the former director general of the World Health Organization, recognised the unique position of health care professionals, especially nurses and midwives, in the promotion of primary preventive health care. He went on to suggest that they take up the challenge and ensure that health care is delivered satisfactorily and effectively. In order for this to come about they must be able to exert the necessary pressure on local and central government to ensure the provision of health education, proper nutrition, safe water, basic sanitation and adequate housing in addition to the preventive, curative and rehabilitative services that the health service already provides.

 Activities

- Explain what is meant by the term 'a universal service'.
- Discuss the differences between collective and individual responsibility.
- Organise a seminar to discuss what is meant by the terms equal and equitable.

REFERENCES

Brown M, Payne S 1994 Introduction to social administration in Britain. Routledge, London

Clarke J, Cochrane A, McLaughlin E 1994 Managing social policy. Sage

Department of Health 1991 The patient's charter. HMSO, London

Klein R 1983 The politics of the National Health Service. Longman, London

McCarthy M 1990 The politics of welfare: an agenda for the 1990s. Macmillan, London

Spicker P 1995 Social policy themes and approaches. Prentice Hall/Harvester Wheatsheaf, Hemel Hempstead

Titmuss R 1963 Essays on the welfare state. Allen and Quinn, London

1

Contextual issues

The emergence of health and social care services in the United Kingdom has been slow in comparison to other public services. The slower pace has, however, helped to ensure that developments have tended to improve the quality and distribution of services. This section will provide the student with historical insight into the social and political circumstances that either coerced or facilitated government to introduce the services we recognise and probably take for granted today.

The development of health and social care services

Kevin Gormley

At the end of this chapter the student should be able to:

- **describe early health and social services provision**
- **discuss the reasons for the poor law and its later amendment**
- **reflect on the role of influential individuals in terms of emerging health and social policy**
- **discuss the reasons why public health services developed**
- **trace the early development of national health and social care services**

Introduction

Any examination of the evolution of government policy towards the provision of health and social services in the early part of the 19th century needs to address three issues. First it must address why government did not or could not provide an appropriate and comprehensive service as of right for all of the nation's citizens, particularly those who had fallen on hard times. Second, the debate must provide an insight into the principle of deterrence that underlined government interventions. Third, interventions by government should be considered in terms of their overall contribution towards the future evolution of health and social services.

Britain has a long history of offering some form of assistance for the sick, destitute and poverty-stricken. As far back as Anglo-Saxon times alms giving was considered to be a central part of religious duty that enabled the ecclesiastics to provide relief for those in need. From the 13th century onwards there was a steady increase in secular involvement, although the role of the religious continued to be the most influential. The reasons for the first movements towards secularism were twofold. First there was a desire among those living in towns and villages to have more control in the distribution of their charitable endowments, and second there was a specific need for greater organisation and authority in order to suppress the increasing problem of vagrancy.

Between the 16th and the 18th centuries Britain expanded politically, economically, socially and intellectually. A renaissance also occurred in universities with the encouragement of creative thinking. This permeated into medical education, which had slowly made its way into the universities, and led to a period of sensitive enlightenment towards developing services for the sick. Ideas of compassion and assistance became entwined with the quest for furthering scientific knowledge. However, this period also witnessed the effects of another movement in Britain, the Reformation, which began in the 16th century as a demand for reform within the church but ended as a revolt, causing an irreversible schism within Christianity. In Britain, the Catholic religious orders were suppressed and, along with them went their responsibilities for caring for the disadvantaged. In ordering the closure of monasteries Henry VIII effectively wiped out most of the existing caring services. The orphaned, the aged, the sick and the dispossessed were left without any provision and without any prospect of a replacement.

Following the abrupt discontinuation of the services provided by religious communities many died from malnutrition while others resorted to begging, which quickly became an offence, often resulting in mutilating punishments. Hospital care also stagnated and services fell into disrepute because of the squalor of the environment and the inadequacy of the staff. As a replacement for the monasteries municipal hospital and alms houses were developed in major towns. These were funded and supported by a combination of individual donation and the benevolence of local industries. However, because of the ad hoc nature of their organisation, neither of these two arrangements were satisfactory. They were merely a reaction to the underlying problem of poverty and the associated effects of ill-health and dependence (Dolan 1973).

EARLY HEALTH CARE SERVICES

The health care needs of the population were met through four discrete forms of service (Box 2.1). First there was a range of practitioners such as barber–surgeons, bone setters and midwives, performing their own specialised forms of treatment. Second, there were cruder forms of public health service dealing with areas such as vermin control or the maintenance of water supplies. These services were often overseen by local magistrates and funded from local taxation. Third, there was assistance provided by church charities such as alms houses and early forms of hospital for the chronically disabled, the poor, the widowed and the orphaned, although this form of service steadily decreased in power and influence with the rise in secularism. The fourth and largest provider of service, as it still is today, was the informal network of friends and family supporting their dependants without any form of outside intervention. Outside of this,

---

Box 2.1 Early health care services

- Specialist practitioners
- Public health services
- Charitable services
- Family support

Activities

- List the early problems of providing a reasonable health and social service in Britain.
- Consider with your colleagues what care would have been like if you were to require surgery during the 16th century.

the well-off were able to pay for private consultations with the growing number of qualified physicians who had received formal university medical training in the universities (Bruce 1974).

Industrialisation

The end of the 18th century was a particularly significant period of economic growth and brought increasing industrialisation. The so-called 'Industrial Revolution' in Britain was not a precise event; its early development began in about 1760 and activity peaked by the 1840s (Hobsbawm 1985). By this time Britain's massive heavy industry, along with its recently-developed railway system, which provided a perfect infrastructure, had created the world's first mature and stable industrial economy. Industrialisation stimulated entrepreneurs towards further technological development and many medical discoveries.

Alongside this, industrialisation also fostered a revolutionary change towards the creation of new political, economic and sociological ideologies. Technological progress affected the means of production and had a particular impact on agriculture. Power-driven machinery replaced the traditional need for human skills and effort. The resulting increase in rural unemployment led to a substantial movement of people to the new cities, bringing urbanisation on an unprecedented scale, and leading to further social problems among the new town dwellers, such as widespread and enduring poverty, overcrowding and disease (Table 2.1).

Previously, when production had been based largely on cottage industries, rural labourers were able to combine light manufacturing work

with farming. On moving to the city this manufacturing class became the hired hands and, more important, were exposed to market forces. Even at a simple level, workers had to pay rent from their wages for accommodation and thus city dwellers became totally dependent on their ability to work and on the availability of employment. Given this new pressure to bring in money, whole households were expected to work and contribute financially, including mothers and young children.

Activity

Discuss with your colleagues the net effects of industrialisation on the provision of health care.

THE POOR

The first recorded statute for the national control of the poor was the Ordinance of Labourers, 1349. This legislation made it illegal for individuals to offer relief to the able-bodied poor on the grounds that everybody should be compelled to labour for their living. This early legislation was of historical importance because for the first time a differentiation was made between sympathetically meeting the needs of the deserving poor and forcing the lazy to become self-reliant. Leonard (1965) contends that the first major reorganisation of poor relief into a recognisable system began during the Tudor period. From the middle of the 16th century to the early years of the following century a series of parliamentary changes were enacted to overhaul the nature of services for the poor and needy. According to Leonard, widespread unemployment led to large numbers of men roaming around and committing a range of crimes to the annoyance and fear of the local community.

Sir Robert Cecil, an influential parliamentarian at the time, articulated the difficulties that faced the poor. Cecil argued that when individuals, through no fault of their own, became unemployed and penniless they had no option but to move around in an attempt to find work. Yet in

Table 2.1	Industrialisation and urbanisation
Entrepreneurial spirit	Loss of cottage industries
Economic prosperity	Loss of individual autonomy
Employment	Poverty
Improved infrastructure (railways)	Overcrowding and homelessness
Medical discoveries	Disease
Early education and health services	Poor working conditions

doing so they risked being whipped or worse because of the fear that vagrants aroused within the settled community. He suggested that a comprehensive and centralised programme was required to tackle the widespread incidence of poverty. This programme included the provision of accommodation for the poor and destitute with the requirement that they undertake community work to avoid idleness. Although they were first described as houses of correction they were in fact an embryo of the workhouse system.

The Poor Law

The Elizabethan Poor Law of 1601, now generally known as the Old Poor Law, was the end stage of a process of failed attempts to quell the problem of poverty. It marked the beginning of a regime which, with slight variations, would last for over 200 years. It also became the cornerstone upon which more stringent systems were developed and the key influence in care provision throughout the British Isles. The Poor Law Act made each parish responsible for those of its own parishioners who had become impoverished, frail or handicapped. The funding for this service was collected via a revised local tax that was administered through a means test calculated by an appointed overseer, later to be referred to as the Relieving Officer.

Subsistence was provided for the needy through either money ('outdoor relief') or various forms of institutional care ('indoor relief'). The former was a benefit offered to people who were temporarily unemployed because of the seasonal nature of some types of work, or it could be used to fund the cost of a physician to attend to the needs of the sick. Indoor relief was provided in three forms for different classifications of pauper. The impotent poor (the chronically sick, the aged, the blind or the mentally ill) were accommodated in poorhouses. The able-bodied were placed in workhouses and were expected to undertake menial labouring jobs. Finally, the able-bodied who persistently absconded and refused to undertake any form of work were placed in houses of correction. This last form of institution was a punishment for idleness

and was administered under a strict and disciplinary regime (Frazer 1984). Although being 'on the parish' was associated with some degree of shame, the only alternative was to enter the parish poorhouse. White (1978) argues that this was not as bad as it seems because according to his records some poorhouses were quite homely.

Little changed after the original 1601 act although there were some later amendments. The Gilbert Act (1782) recommended that parish workhouses should combine to form unions with an infirmary where the sick and aged could receive more humane or appropriate care. Former workhouses and Gilbert unions varied greatly in structure and management. Some of the smaller ones were old farmhouses in need of considerable repair while others were so large and impressive they were locally referred to as pauper palaces. In the case of the former, Longmate (1974) suggests that conditions were so bad it was open to speculation 'whether the worn out inmate would survive his wretched hovel or it him'. The great majority of workhouses were relatively lax in terms of discipline and open to abuse in that the standard of living often exceeded that of the rate-paying and working labourer. The situation was made worse during periods of economic downturn because of the increasing numbers of able-bodied people resorting to indoor support.

Activities

- Make a list of the reasons why poverty was a major problem for 17th-century Britain.
- Discuss with your friends why it was a difficult problem to resolve.

The Poor Law Amendment Act

Criticism levelled against the Elizabethan poor law was partly economic and partly moral. The total expenditure on the poor rose rapidly, particularly in the period between 1815 and 1830. The cost, it was claimed, placed an unjust burden on the predominantly middle-class rate-payers who had to fund welfare through local property taxes (Williams 1981). Apart from being unjust, it was thought that high rates stifled economic development. Conversely, it was also believed that high benefits encouraged idleness. From a moral perspective it was claimed that poor law relief discouraged thrift and personal independence, thereby undermining the sanctity of the family.

Background

At the beginning of the 19th century Britain was one of the most powerful economic states in the world. Despite this relatively halcyon period, a sizeable proportion of the population was likely to experience poverty at some time in their lives. Even the higher skilled and higher paid artisans of the time frequently found themselves out of work due to economic downturns. In these circumstances household incomes were dependent either on credit or on money earned by wives or children.

Liberal economists of the time were not overly concerned with transitory or temporary poverty, the argument being that, although unfortunate, it was a necessary element for the maintenance of a natural economic order. It was believed that exposure to these difficult circumstances inspired people to work, thus preventing similar economic circumstances from arising again. The main concern at this time was the rising level of pauperism and the cost of maintaining the existing poor law, particularly the system of outdoor relief.

The attitude of the general public to pauperism was a combination of the fatalistic (there is nothing that can be done) and the moralistic (pauperism is the result of individual weakness of character). Midwinter (1994) reported that in 1832 there were 1.5 million paupers in England and Wales, or approximately 10% of the total population. It was not surprising that in any review of the Elizabethan poor law, the revision of the system of outdoor relief payments was an important factor. When the Royal Commission on the Poor Law conducted an inquiry in 1832/33 it was understood from the outset that the commission's members were appointed to

provide an alternative to the payment of outdoor relief.

The Royal Commission dispatched assistant commissioners to visit parishes all around the country and report back on the various ways in which the existing poor law worked in each area. Even at this stage there were accusations that assistant commissioners were liberals and were therefore selective in the areas that they visited. Frazer (1984) suggests that they were careful only to report situations that reiterated their concerns in regard to abuses of outdoor relief. It would be fair to suggest that the eventual report, published in 1834, was principally aimed at deterring pauperism rather than reducing poverty.

When the government received the report from the Royal Commission it quickly enacted the Poor Law Amendment Act, 1834, which contained most of its major points (see Box 2.2),

---

Box 2.2 Main recommendations of the Poor Law Report 1834

- Centralisation: all control of caring services for the poor and dependent would be from the central board of control. Local overseers would remain in place but they would be accountable to the new Board.
- The workhouse test: this was a self-assessment test of destitution. The only relief to be provided for the able-bodied would be the offer of a place in a workhouse. Outdoor relief was not abolished but was substantially reduced, although provision for medical attendance was maintained. Those who were genuinely in need of assistance would, it was anticipated, either have to accept the harsh regime of a union workhouse or die of starvation.
- Uniformity: for the first time the care provided would be exactly the same, irrespective of where it was offered. This ended the need for the Elizabethan acts of settlement, wherein theoretically paupers were returned to their place of birth to receive support. It also eliminated the considerable variation in services that previously existed, where relatively well-off and charitable areas tended to have better services than poorer districts.
- Classification: there would be a single system of institutional accommodation for able-bodied paupers, and males and females would be separated, as would the young, the old and the handicapped.
- The principle of less eligibility: it was agreed that conditions in the workhouse for the pauper in terms of diet and living arrangements would be continuously monitored and they must at all times be at a level of less than the lowest independent worker.

the most important of which was the principle of eligibility.

Principle of less eligibility

The principle of 'less eligibility' was introduced because the Commission argued that any form of state welfare interfered with an individual's work ethic and the need for private thrift. The principle also underlined the Commission's attempt to substitute the workhouse as an alternative to outdoor relief for able-bodied paupers (Checkland & Checkland 1974, Williams 1981). Incarceration in a workhouse was only considered as being preferable to the alternative of letting the poor and destitute starve. This was not out of humanistic or altruistic concern, but rather to ensure social control and to minimise the risk of criminal acts from potentially desperate and hungry paupers.

Jordan (1974) suggests that the workhouse system was also about creating a mechanism for separating the incorrigible or lazy from the more industrious poor. The latter were encouraged by government through various social reforms to be loyal and good citizens while the former were simply institutionalised. Thus political control was maintained. Furthermore, in creating these two classifications it was argued that the taint of pauperism would not be able to infect the honest working man. This underlined the Victorian belief that pauperism was a combination of self-inflicted circumstances that could be transferred to others. This double-edged caring and deterrent strategy towards dealing with the poor survived for nearly 80 years.

Activities

- Outline the reasons for the Poor Law Amendment Act.
- Discuss with your colleagues the purpose of this legislation.
- Organise a debate to discuss value of the Poor Law Amendment Act.

The effects of poverty

Marshall (1967) contends that to understand the extent of poverty in 19th-century Britain one must consider the net sociological effect of having been labelled a pauper. This was not just a reflection of an individual's inability to provide housing, food or clothing – being a pauper implied accepting a status of second-class citizenship, a status that was extended to include his family. The term pauper implied an underclass with the resultant loss of any previous good standing or reputation. Ultimately it meant the giving up of all rights and personal freedom through an automatic disenfranchisement and detention in a workhouse. The comprehensive character of the status of pauper meant that other essential services such as health care or education, were provided separately, and only to those in similar social circumstances. The pauper's health was attended to by the appointed poor law medical officer or, if necessary, by the infirmary, and children of pauper families were sent to poor law schools. Impoverished people were intentionally caught in the trap of social indignity and stigma, with only the veil of a pauper's grave to look forward to.

Activity

Make brief notes and then form a group to discuss the purpose of the principle of ineligibility.

The poor law and older people

Social concern about the treatment of the old and infirm within the workhouse had prevailed from the very beginning of the implementation of the 1834 Act. Repeated efforts to afford concessions were regularly defeated because of the fear that 'pampering' special groups would permeate the establishment and undermine the workhouse as a deterrent to pauperism. The 1833 Royal Commission did recommend that 'the old might enjoy their indulgences', however, there is little evidence to suggest any allowances were made. In 1842 the Poor Law Commissioners informed unions that workhouse uniforms were not compulsory but this went unheeded. Inmates in the workhouse were not supposed to have personal belongings of any sort, therefore there was no need for personal lockers. The absence of any chairs meant paupers had only their beds to sit on or benches in the yard. Even the inner window sills were deliberately sloped to avoid their use as a seat or shelf. It was 1890 before the aged and other 'deserving paupers' were allowed to receive gifts of sweets, dry tea or tobacco (Longmate 1974, Pinker 1979, Rose 1986).

There was an economic up-turn in the second half of the 19th century and the period was marked by stirrings of reform. An increase in personal wealth and prosperity contributed to a fall in the number of able-bodied residents in workhouses. The effects of this change were offset by a corresponding increase in the number of dependent people entering the workhouse who were in need of some form of nursing care. This was demonstrated by visits to 39 London unions by the *Lancet*'s Sanitary Commission (1865), who were investigating the state of workhouse infirmaries. Out of a total of 31 000 inmates only 2300 (7.4%) were considered to be fit and able to work.

Old age, coupled with disease or long term disability, had become the chief reason for people resorting to the status of paupers (Norton 1988, Pinker 1964). As a result of these investigations it was apparent that workhouses were rapidly becoming infirmaries for frail and dependent individuals. Largely through the work of reformers such as physicians Joseph Rogers and Louis Twining, the Lancet Commission and a number of influential lay people, humanitarian principles gradually took hold and led to a wave of major reform. The first serious moral challenge came from Beatrice Webb in the Minority

Activities

- List five reasons why it was difficult for the government at the time to separate the deserving and undeserving poor.
- Discuss the value of these reasons.

Report on the Commission of the Poor Laws in 1909. She advocated that responsibility for the non-able-bodied, including the elderly, children and the long term sick, should be transferred from the poor law to local authorities and central government preventive services.

INFLUENTIAL INDIVIDUALS

Marshall (1966) contends that much of the momentum for change in early 19th-century social policy can be directly attributed to the determined efforts of key individuals. These men, who were mainly doctors or civil servants, were able to exert more political influence than the collective power of either local or central government. They had immense courage, energy and outstanding ability and were labelled as the pioneers of the great advance.

Adam Smith

The 18th century is often referred to as the Age of Enlightenment. It was a time of optimism, particularly among scholars who strove to provide a new social order. Philosophers such as Adam Ferguson and the Marquis de Condorcet used their analyses of social progress to provide indicators or directions for further growth and development. Adam Smith was strongly influenced by their thoughts and sought to provide new laissez-faire ideas that would act as underpinnings for continued economic growth, development and prosperity. As the population of Britain moved further away from royal subject status towards citizenship, new ideas began to evolve that would create further freedom and liberty. Smith was a convert towards policies that encouraged individualism and enterprise. To this end he was opposed to excessive government intervention as a means of solving societal problems such as poverty or universal health care.

The social argument of Adam Smith's philosophy was that humanity was essentially about the rights of individuals to be free to choose, to take the lead in their own destiny and to compete with one another. If these human features were left unchecked, which he favoured, they would ultimately produce a natural order which would present as a division of labour. In other words, there was a need for the existence of a class of capitalists owning the means of production and a labouring class supporting them in their growth. Both groups, Smith argued, were mutually dependent on each other and together they could provide the means for stimulating continuous economic growth. In his classic publication, *The Wealth of Nations* (1776), Smith laid the economic foundations of utilitarianism. Smith argued that leaving the market to the invisible hand of supply and demand was the best way of creating a natural balance that would meet the needs of the collective and the individual simultaneously. In other words, Smith believed that there was natural balance in the motivation of enterprising individuals between self-seeking and the well-being of society, and that the advancement of industrious persons would lead ultimately to the advancement of everybody.

Midwinter (1994) argues that Smith's doctrine was more opportunistic than realistic: it was reasonable enough for Smith to argue against monitory control during a period when Britain was at its peak as a major economic force, with no serious competitors on the world scene and with a strong navy, an expanding empire, relatively stable political conditions, a sound banking system and a society that fostered the entrepreneurial spirit. Smith's ideas encouraged consecutive governments throughout the first half of the 19th century to minimise their interventions, lest their interference constrict further growth and development. Pinker (1995) describes this period as the golden age of unparalleled individualism, economic growth, burgeoning prosperity and exemplary family values. Pinker does, however, point out that at the same time as Smith's ideas were in the ascendancy the early stirrings of a movement towards socialism were also beginning to be felt. Profit and individual achievement were the watchwords but alongside this there was widespread suffering and destitution, compounded by a poor law that threatened family break up as a further deterrent.

Early social reformers

Smith was not unaware of the needs of the sick and poor but offered little in terms of addressing them, a vacuum that socialist theorists such as Robert Owen, William Thompson and John Gray were quick to fill. They argued that utilitarianism was exploitative and oppressive of the labouring classes. What was needed was a trustworthy form of government that would foster 'co-operative altruism instead of competitive egoism' (Pinker 1995). Hobsbawm (1985) points out that the notion of revolution quickly ferments among the poor if living standards do not rise for all. The early period of socialism, beginning with Robert Owen's *New View of Society* (1813–14) and the launch of the *Communist Manifesto* (1848), Hobsbawm reminds us, was a period of increasing relative depression, with falling wages, high technological unemployment and poor confidence in the potential for expansion in the economy. Early socialists who were opposed to free-market liberalism blamed it for destroying the social order of the traditional community and its inherent capacity for human caring.

Jeremy Bentham

Very few individuals from the 19th century have attracted as much attention among revisionist historians as Jeremy Bentham. A combination of new information and debate among social historians has altered considerably the current views of his influence. To some historians he was a posthumous revolutionary guru, responsible for the creation of the Victorian administrative state. To others he was merely a bit player, responsible for minor administrative changes. What is without doubt, however, is his influential role in three discrete areas. First, in the legal field, he highlighted a need for a comprehensive body of law, an elaborate legal system and a clear division of offences. He wished to create a legislative system that was without blank spaces, in which there was nothing left unprovided for, and a body of law complete in all its branches. Second he was an ardent proponent of Adam Smith's economic philosophy, constantly arguing the case for complete freedom of trade and the need to withdraw from statute any form of paternalism that artificially affected the marketplace. Thirdly he played an important role in social reform, particularly in the area of institutional care for convicts in prisons and paupers in the workhouses.

Bentham died before the new poor law workhouses became operational, nevertheless his views on the role of the state and pauperism were evident. He provided three arguments in justification of a poor law that had an inbuilt support for harshness and degradation. First, Bentham argued, institutions for paupers should be a last resort and be so designed that they would assist individuals in the development of self-reliance and discipline. Second, he believed that the workhouse's behaviourist strategies would be particularly beneficial to children born into the system who, from the outset of their lives, would be indoctrinated by the regime with ideals of personal thrift and self-discipline; this would, in the long term, prevent the inevitability of their continuing their lives as paupers. Third, on a macro level, he believed that individual happiness was linked to self-reliance and the threat of a form of penal servitude in the workhouse, for those opting to become dependent, was a necessary deterrent (Lieberman 1985).

Bentham's projects, although radical, were at the same time a conservative mechanism for reducing social disquiet within Britain. Overall, Bentham's utilitarian philosophy, which was an amalgam of economics, eugenics and behaviourist ideas, seems to have infiltrated public opinion and influenced legislative policy for nearly half a century. For this reason he must be considered in any analysis of the development of social policy in 19th-century Britain. However, it is useful to separate Bentham the person from Benthamism because there is little evidence of major political movement or any revolutionary government policy that can be fully attributed to him.

Seebohm Rowntree and Charles Booth

Benjamin Seebohm Rowntree was the son of the Quaker cocoa manufacturer, philanthropist and pioneer of industrial welfare, Joseph Rowntree. He is regarded as having originated in 1901 a scientific definition of poverty as: 'the minimum income level required for physical subsistence'. He was also a pioneer of social research into poverty. The findings in his first study, published in 1901, not only counted the poor but described their social conditions. This report demonstrated that in spite of all the legislative changes and increases in the living standard of British society, wealth did not naturally percolate down to the labouring classes. Rowntree showed that at least one third of the poor had insufficient money to purchase enough goods even for a satisfactory physical existence (Veit-Wilson 1986).

Briggs (1961) argues that Rowntree's report was a cornerstone in developing a clear understanding of poverty for three reasons. First, it was the first attempt to gauge the extent of national poverty. Second, Rowntree developed a reliable and scientific instrument for measuring poverty and determining a minimum level at which poverty would begin. Third, Rowntree, through his study, inverted the previous belief that poverty was associated with sloth, lifestyle or misuse of sufficient resources. He replaced this concept with a new perspective of poverty as being too little money for a minimum subsistence.

Charles Booth, a wealthy ship owner from Liverpool who had settled in London in the 1870s, was influenced by the social unrest at the time to investigate the true facts about poverty in London. His survey was not intended to provide remedies or explanations for poverty, but rather simply to provide a snapshot of its extent in the capital. The results were broadly similar to Rowntree's in terms of the percentage of the population affected by poverty, the residual effects of overcrowding and squalor, and the correlation between poverty and a high mortality rate. The reports of both Rowntree and Booth also showed that low wages, large families, irregularity of employment and actual unemployment kept an enormous number of people below the poverty line. This last finding paved the way for the setting up of a national insurance scheme in the century that was to follow.

Activities

- Make brief notes on the political ideology of Adam Smith.
- Discuss whether or not Adam Smith has been an influence on 20th-century policy.

POOR LAW AND SOCIAL POLICY

It is usual to associate the name of Edwin Chadwick with the Royal Commission's Poor Law Report, which was published in 1834. This is possibly because history has labelled him as the most influential mover and shaker, but there were in fact eight other commission members: Nassau Senior, Bishop Bloomfield of London, Bishop Sumner of Chester, William Sturges Bourne MP, the Revd Henry Bishop, Henry Gawler, Walter Coulson and James Traill. It was originally argued by historians that because the Poor Law Commission was linked to Chadwick and his co-author Senior, the report was simply a vehicle for furthering Benthamite or utilitarian ideas. It is true that both men were considered as disciples of Jeremy Bentham (Nassau Senior, for example, had assisted in the foundation of the Political Economy Club, a group committed to the utilitarian philosophy and ideals developed by Bentham during the late 18th century). However, what is frequently omitted in debates regarding the poor law is the fact that, except for these two men, all of the remaining members of the commission were either Tory or traditionally Tory supporters.

It is now broadly accepted that the poor law was not particularly revolutionary, nor part of an inspired shift in British political ideology, but rather part of a gradual change which came about as a reaction to many social, political and economic pressures that had previously existed. Mandler (1990) argues that the new Poor Law was a pragmatic combination of liberal and Tory ideas designed in differing ways to suit both groups' traditional ideologies. Mandler concedes that Chadwick and Senior did contribute to an overall reorganisation of rural society towards more liberal ideas where individuals were encouraged to become more self-reliant. This was, however, Tory inspired. Mandler contends that although the paternalistic old poor law was always anathema to the liberals it had also become a millstone for Tory landlords. The revolution in France and, in Britain, rural unsettlement caused by increasing industrialisation, had created new circumstances in which the control of land became an issue. As a result, the protection afforded to the labouring classes which guaranteed their acquiescence and enabled landlords to exert power, influence and control no longer applied. The net effect of this was twofold: the new poor law permitted landlords to jettison their previous responsibilities to protect the labouring classes; however, they were still able to retain power over the labourers through high rents and control of the new markets that had been created.

UNIVERSAL SERVICE

The new poor law

At a societal level the new poor law was designed as a final solution to the problem of pauperism, while for the individual it was interpreted as a rehabilitative mechanism that could help the moral character of the working man. In reality, at both levels, the poor law was clearly nothing of the sort. For residents in the workhouses cruelty, in all its forms, was the order of the day. Within the 600 new workhouses that were built in England and Wales in the first 70 years following the implementation of the Act, harsh and depersonalising regulations were rigidly adhered to by the local boards of guardians (Box 2.3). These included prison-like discipline, strict time-tabling of daily events, the enforced wearing of depersonalising uniforms and, most

---

Box 2.3 Workhouse regime

- Prison-like discipline
- Time-tabling of daily events
- Uniforms
- Separation of families

harsh of all, the separation of families (Batley 1978). The poor law laid down in minute detail the duties of staff and the manner in which they were to be carried out. Nevertheless, Adams (1992) argues, even within such a closely regulated system the wide geographical spread of the poor law made it impossible for conditions to be exactly the same everywhere. Until relatively recently, historians have relied extensively on the literary works of Charles Dickens, for example, to provide a picture of the conditions for paupers in the workhouse.

It is not in dispute that the new poor law created a harsh and bureaucratic hierarchical universal structure within all workhouse environments. The workhouses were correctly satirised as 'Bastilles' in which married couples were separated and the inmates tyrannised by masters like Dickens's domineering fictional beadle, Mr Bumble, in *Oliver Twist*. It is true that the head of the workhouse, the master, was in absolute charge and it was he who set the tone for the administration of the workhouse and provided guidance for the behaviour of subordinate staff. Adams (1992) does, however, take issue with the notion that all masters behaved in the manner of Mr Bumble or that all paupers were treated like Oliver Twist. Gutchen (1984) too suggests that too often the historical evidence is either distorted or ignored in favour of fictional characters or factual scandals which, while true, were not necessarily a reflection of the national picture. Gutchen provides significant evidence to argue two key points. First, within many workhouses masters displayed a great deal of sensitivity to the needs of their charges in terms of promoting their welfare and encouraging a family atmosphere among the staff. Second, it could be argued that masters of workhouses played a positive role in the evolution process of the welfare state. This view would be in contrast to the more simplistic argument that the harsh conditions of the workhouse created the momentum for substantive reform of services for the poor and the eventual evolution of the welfare state. What is without doubt, however, is that the poor law reaffirmed the principle that the state had a responsibility to ensure some basic standard of livelihood for its citizens and from that standard developed most of our modern programmes of public welfare.

The poor law was an abject failure in terms of its attempt to combine the separate concepts of deterrence and compassion. For these reasons the Poor Law Amendment Act, 1834, will probably always be associated with fear and hatred and known as a piece of legislation that did a great disservice to those members of society who were most in need, the old, the poor and the handicapped. Conversely, it should be remembered that the 1834 Act was also, at the same time, a bench-mark for the notion of state involvement in that it was the first government attempt at implementing a national or universal social policy. Whatever its failings and despite its harshness, the Poor Law Amendment Act, in historical terms, has been recognised as a forerunner to the provision of National Assistance in many areas such as old age pensions, supplementary benefits, family allowance and the National Health Service.

Local authorities

Although the 1834 Poor Law Amendment Act has been described as radical in terms of the centralisation of authority, it is important to point out that local authorities remained a powerful force in its implementation. In addition, many of the Act's key proposals were already in existence. The original act, for instance, suggested that individual parishes should unite to form larger unions, so that parish institutional services could be replaced by larger and more cost-effective single union poorhouses. This had already happened in many parts of the country following the enactment of the Gilbert Act, 1782. As to the question of outdoor relief, the changes were met with a great deal of opposition from around the country and outdoor relief was never fully abolished. Indeed, there was so much hostility that the Poor Law Commission agreed to permit continued outdoor payments provided some attempt was made by the recipient to engage in some form of labour or employment.

Activity

Discuss with your teacher whether the Poor Law was an antagonist or part of the process leading towards a welfare state.

PHILANTHROPISTS

Philanthropy has been defined as the desire to do good to others, particularly when this involves direct contact between donor and recipient and the provision of such services within a sensitive relationship. Roach (1978) describes Lord Ashley, the seventh Earl of Shaftesbury, as both the greatest and most characteristic of the philanthropists because of his deep involvement in a range of causes, including the humane treatment of the mentally ill, reform of the factory acts and the endemic problem of poverty, particularly in the inner cities. Shaftesbury was an untypical member of the landed gentry in many ways; firstly because of the unusual degree of compassion he felt towards the disadvantaged as a whole, not confining his charitable instincts to his tenantry as many landlords did. Secondly, in spite of his title and land he was a comparatively poor man, who inherited significant debts on the death of his father. Despite this, all of his positions on various boards were unpaid. Other influential 19th-century philanthropic activities included Octavia Hill's housing experiments, Beatrice Webb's pressure for prison reform, General Booth's Salvation Army and Florence Nightingale's work in developing a professional nursing service for the sick.

Collectivism versus individualism

As health and social services developed throughout the 19th century there was a degree of tension between two contrasting philosophies of welfare provision, collectivism and individualism (state action through the intervention of local authorities or central government as against private initiative by means of personal philanthropy). The need for public education

programmes addressing issues such as hygiene and cleanliness highlights the ideological debate between collective and individual action that existed at the time and continues to the present. Radical reformers argued that public health was directly influenced by a combination of environmental and social conditions and required community or government accountability for its enforcement. In spite of this, the beginnings of sanitary reform can be traced to early philanthropists and intellectuals from the middle classes, such as Florence Nightingale. The earliest form of a recognisable health visiting service, in Manchester and Salford in the 1860s, began as a group of middle class women collectively trying to meet the health needs of the poor through education about hygiene and sanitation (Dingwall 1977).

Philanthropy versus mutual aid or self-help

Jones (1993) contextualises philanthropy by contrasting its role with alternative forms of action such as mutual aid or personal thrift. Mutual aid addresses the attempts of working men to protect each other against inevitable crises of their lives (such as illness, unemployment, disability or old age) through the setting up of trade unions or associations to organise insurance and safer working conditions. Personal thrift, or self-help, was about taking responsibility and making provision for oneself. Much of the ideals associated with personal thrift are linked with the ideology of Samuel Smiles (1884), who optimistically believed that 19th-century Britain was an earlier form of meritocracy. Through hard work, Smiles argued, it was possible for the working man to achieve anything. He did not argue that the potential for upwards social movement or increased economic wealth necessarily existed for everybody, although the early entrepreneurs were possible examples of this. He was instead suggesting that it was possible for the labouring man to be an individual free to develop new ideas and appreciate the aesthetic aspects of life. To this end he wrote, 'any class of man that lives from hand to mouth will forever be an inferior class, hanging on to the skirts of society', and advocated the provision of free public libraries, education and museums. It was the doctrine of encouraging thrift, or prepare-for-a-rainy-day mentality, that prompted the setting up of a wide range of accessible commercial institutions including building societies, friendly societies and post office savings banks.

Activities

- List five ways in which philanthropists assisted the poor and needy in society.
- Consider the motivations of philanthropists and discuss with your colleagues their value.

PUBLIC HEALTH SERVICES

Sanitation

Apart from the poor law amendment, one of the most important areas of government health policy was the provision of public health services that were created to promote the prevention of disease. Throughout the 19th century infectious diseases such as cholera and typhoid posed a major threat to the general population. Medical intervention was at this time largely powerless to intervene because little was understood about the nature of disease. Although normally only the most poverty-stricken areas of towns were affected, particularly virulent epidemics swept through whole communities, affecting both rich and poor. While home conditions were obviously bad for most people, the situation at work was even worse. Most factories employed large numbers of people in buildings that had poor ventilation, no sunlight and miserable hygiene facilities. Within these insanitary conditions diseases such as cholera were able to find a strong foothold. The cumulative effect of these poor conditions, along with the effects of poor quality of food and inadequate sewerage systems, prompted the government to set up boards of health. Early health boards instituted strict cleansing regimes during cholera outbreaks and also provided soup kitchens.

The agreed reason for the eventual substantial decrease in the incidence and severity of diseases such as cholera and typhoid was the development of a public health system. A major influence in the Royal Commission was Edwin Chadwick, whose *Report of an Inquiry into the Sanitary Conditions of the Labouring Population of Great Britain in 1842* prompted the government's introduction of the 1848 Public Health Act. This Act ensured the adequate supply of water and sewerage systems and provided for the formation of a centralised General Board of Health. Even mundane services such as the burial of the dead came under the remit of the public health services.

Hospital services

During the 18th century ever increasing numbers of people moved from their agrarian bases to the new industrial cities, whose populations were rapidly increasing. The population of Bristol, for example, rose from 20 000 to 60 000, Glasgow from 13 000 to 80 000. Manchester, by 1801, had trebled its size to approximately 85 000 in less than 25 years. These demographic changes, along with the growth of university-trained doctors, allowed for the creation of new voluntary hospitals in many British cities. Funding for these came from a combination of contributions from local industry and charitable organisations. The first such hospital to be opened, the Westminster in London, was quickly followed by similar establishments in Edinburgh, Bristol, York and Liverpool.

Voluntary hospitals made a valuable contribution to health care. They were, however, far from the ideal model. In the first instance they operated on a privileged system of patronage in that the sick were required to bring a letter of recommendation from a subscriber to the hospital in order to gain admission. Second, voluntary hospitals did not provide services for maternity care, sick children, the dying, or people with tuberculosis, epilepsy, syphilis or any other infectious disease. The only form of institutional service for these people was in the workhouse infirmaries.

Hospital services did begin to improve by

the middle of the 19th century. The voluntary hospitals developed closer affinities with medical faculties in universities and care was gradually extended. The number of beds within each hospital increased and out-patient departments evolved, in which patients could be properly assessed and accurate reviews made of their progress. Nevertheless, care in hospital continued to focus on acute and treatable conditions, creating pressure for specialist hospitals. As a result new specialist services emerged, including new institutions catering for maternity care, sick children, eyes and particular diseases.

For patients with infectious diseases or certain chronic conditions, for whom the workhouse infirmary remained the only alternative, conditions were harsh, largely because of the degree of overcrowding and poor hygiene within these institutions. The medical profession exerted constant pressure for change and improvement. Significant improvements were achieved following the enactment of the 1867 Metropolitan Poor Act which allowed for the development of new infirmaries in London that were separate from the workhouse system. This policy was later extended to the rest of the country within the 1868 Poor Law Amendment Act. At about the same time public dispensaries and rudimentary health centres were also being developed. Ham (1985) contends that the combined effect of these two programmes was an important step in English economic and social history, particularly the provision of infirmaries, since this was the first explicit acknowledgement by government of its responsibility to provide a form of health service for the poor which did not, at the same time, threaten retribution or the punishment of a workhouse.

Mental health care

Hospital services for the mentally ill evolved in a slightly different way to other health services in Britain. By the turn of the 19th century there were two forms of provision. There were private madhouses which operated as profit-making businesses, providing a service for those who could afford such provision. In addition, approval had been given to local counties to build county asylums for people with mental health problems. However, due to a lack of available funds and of motivation within the authorities, very few were actually built in the first decades of the century. People in need of mental health services either remained at home or, if that was not possible, they were accommodated along with the old, sick or homeless as inmates in the poor law workhouses or with criminals in gaols. With the passing of the 1845 Lunatics Act every county was compelled to provide purpose-built accommodation for the mentally ill, thus enabling the decanting and, at the same time, reclassification of large numbers of poor law paupers. It was originally intended that the milieu of these new asylums would focus on treatment and maximising the potential of cure for patients. The provision of in-patient services was supposed to be interpreted as a period of retreat or natural time out. None of this ever materialised. Even the idea that asylums should be small buildings offering the equivalent of a homely and family support network was quickly jettisoned. As new asylums were built they correspondingly increased in size, so much so that by the turn of the 20th century the average population of each asylum had risen from 100 to 1000 (for further information see Chapter 10).

Conclusion

This chapter has highlighted the increase in central control over those areas of social policy that affect public health and well-being. Although most of these developments were implemented in the first three decades of the 19th century, it has been shown that the first movements towards change probably began in the preceding half century. Furthermore, any changes that were enacted proved, for the most part, to be merely a framework for action and fell short of a system that would continue to evolve well into the 20th century. The chapter has also acknowledged the strong moralistic beliefs that underpinned attitudes to evolving health and social care policies. In addition, it has described how reforms and reformers shared an ideological philosophy to which Adam Smith and, later, Jeremy Bentham probably contributed, but whose implementation was much more broad based. The success of the development of these services, irrespective of the debate as to whether or not they were satisfactory, must be gauged against the historical backdrop of revolutions and other civil unrest in the rest of the developed world, much of which has been aimed at improving the lot of the less well off members of society as well as at the goal of political independence.

By the end of the 19th century the age-old problem of ad hoc services, where some districts were poorly provided with services in comparison to others, was considered to be intolerable. The trend for national standards of health and services had become firmly rooted in all spheres of British society. Over the previous century changes had occurred not only within governments but also in public attitudes. The doctrine

of individualism, independence and personal control of destiny was no longer considered a complete answer. Although it had always been obvious that some people were unable, for a variety of reasons, to fend for themselves, people now realised that, in some spheres, municipal or government responsibility was more appropriate than private action to meet the needs of everyone.

Activities

- Discuss what living conditions would have been like during the 19th century, in the absence of the public health services that we take for granted today.
- Consider with your teacher which development was more important: the provision of hospitals or effective sanitary and public hygiene services and discuss the reasons why.

REFERENCES

Adams J 1992 Master and matron: work and marriage in the public institution history of nursing. Society Journal 4(3):125–130

Batley R 1978 From poor law to positive discrimination. Journal of Social Policy 7(3):305–328

Briggs A 1961 Social thought and social action: a study of the work of Sebohm Rowntree. Longman, Harlow

Bruce M 1974 The coming of the welfare state. Batsford, London

Checkland S G, Checkland E O (eds) 1974 The Poor Law Report of 1834. Penguin, Harmondsworth

Dingwall R 1977 Collectivism, regionalism and feminism: health visiting and British policy, 1850–1957. Journal of Social Policy 6(3):291–315

Dolan J 1973 Nursing in society: a historical perspective. Saunders, London

Frazer D 1984 The evolution of the British welfare state, 2nd edn. Macmillan, London

Gutchen R M 1984 Masters of workhouses under the poor law. The Local Historian 16(2):93–99 (Cited in Adams 1992)

Ham C 1985 Health policy in Britain. Macmillan, London

Hobsbawm E J 1985 The age of revolution, 1789–1848. Abacus, London

Jones K 1993 The making of social policy in Britain, 1830–1990. Athlone Press, London

Jordan B 1974 Poor parents: social policy and the 'cycle of deprivation'. Routledge and Kegan Paul, London

Leonard E M 1965 The early history of English poor relief. Cass, London

Lieberman D (1985) Historical review from Bentham to Benthamism. Historical Journal 28,1,199–224

Longmate N 1974 The workhouse. Temple-Smith, London (Cited in Norton 1988)

Mandler P 1990 Tories and paupers: Christian political economy and the making of the new poor law. Historical Journal 33(Mar):81–103

Marshall T H 1967 Social policy in the twentieth century. Hutchinson, London

Midwinter E 1994 The development of social welfare in Britain. Open University, Milton Keynes

Norton D 1988 The age of old age. Scutari, London

Pinker R A 1979 The idea of welfare. Heinemann, London

Pinker R A 1964 English hospital statistics. Heinemann, London

Pinker R A 1995 Golden ages and welfare alchemists. Social Policy and Administration 29(2):78–90

Roach J 1978 Social reform in England, 1780–1880. St Martin's Press, New York

Rose M E 1986 The relief of poverty. Macmillan, London

Smiles S 1884 Self help; with illustrations of conduct and perseverance (Cited in Roach 1978)

Veit-Wilson J H 1986 Paradigms of poverty: a rehabilitation of Seebohm Rowntree. Journal of Social Policy 15(1):69–99

White R 1978 Social change and the development of the nursing profession: study of the poor law nursing service, 1848–1948. Kimpton, London

Williams K 1981 From pauperism to poverty. Routledge, London

3

The NHS and the welfare state

Kevin Gormley

At the end of this chapter the student will be able to:

- appreciate the concept of the welfare state and the reasons why it was introduced
- describe the services that emerged as part of the welfare state
- discuss the principles that underlined the welfare state
- trace the evolution of the NHS as a component of the welfare state
- consider the political processes that influenced the NHS
- describe the organisational arrangements of the early NHS
- appreciate the early problems of the NHS

Introduction

In June 1941 Sir William Beveridge, a liberal economist, was appointed to chair an inter-departmental committee on social insurance and allied services. This committee produced a report in December 1942 proposing a comprehensive scheme of social security and also a matching health service that would be accessible and equally comprehensive. The Ministry for Reconstruction, an interim wartime cabinet department, accepted the proposals contained in the Beveridge Report and advised the war cabinet to plan for a health service covering all forms of preventive and curative care. This was endorsed by the cabinet and officially announced in February 1943 (Owen 1988, Webster 1988). As a result the wartime coalition government immediately opened negotiations with existing health and social service providers.

THE BEGINNINGS OF A WELFARE STATE

During the war, the political concept of a fairer system of social welfare and a comprehensive health service became bound up with the broader aims of reconstructing Britain when hostilities ceased. Politicians broadly agreed that there was a need to bring about a more secure and egalitarian society, although the means of achieving this objective differed between the three main political parties. The landslide victory for the Labour Party in the 1945 general election provided an opportunity for the implementation of policies that were not, however, necessarily socialist in origin.

Previously the government had tended to ignore many of the imbalances that existed between population groups and geographical areas, which included:

- the disproportionate distribution of unemployment
- the impact on specific regions and industries
- the inaccessibility of public services to disadvantaged groups
- employees who had occupational insurance were covered against unemployment, sickness and old age, whereas uninsured workers were not.

Effects of the Second World War

Generally, for the marginalised within society in the early 20th century the poor law had been the only public provision (Fraser 1984). The emerging philosophy, which was evident in the Beveridge Report, and the resultant legislative changes fostered an ethos of collective responsibility and action. This was in contrast to the utilitarian doctrine that had been the leading influence on government hitherto (see Chapter 2). There were a number of reasons for this but the most influential was the social and economic upheaval brought about by the Second World War (Timmins 1996).

Social effects

The war was a new experience for the general population in that the effects were more extensive and indiscriminate than those of any previous conflict. Previous wars had mostly been fought far from Britain, and the people at home had not been directly affected. This time everybody had to endure food rationing, and the evacuation of children and bombing of urban conurbations were widespread. As well as this, the total population potentially required emergency medical services and safe shelter. This common experience produced a widespread political spirit that was transferred into a desire for extensive social change (Marshall 1967).

Economic and structural effects

Apart from the devastation resulting from the Second World War, it also had some predictable and possible economic effects, each of which created a degree of pressure for reform in health and welfare provision. First it absorbed unemployment, thereby maximising the potential for public contributions, and at the same time minimised the demand for welfare benefits. Second, it stimulated health services, particularly in an organisational sense, to meet the expected increase in wartime casualties. Third, large amounts of any existing housing stock which had been deemed to be sub-standard was razed. As a result, an extensive rebuilding programme was instituted which significantly improved the living conditions of citizens, particularly in the inner city areas. The legacy of the war was also significant in so far as it created an economic climate that was conducive to implementing many of the policies contained in the Beveridge Report. As well as being able to restore old trade links with the commonwealth countries, new markets were created as many other countries commenced reconstruction work.

Activities

- List five reasons why the welfare state was introduced.
- Consider with your colleagues what it must have been like to live and work in Britain without the protection of the welfare state.

A WELFARE STATE

The welfare state that evolved in Britain was the end product of a radical programme of policies which had been translated from a range of philosophical principles. This was in contrast to the ad hoc and piecemeal services that had been slowly introduced during the preceding 50 years. It was also an attempt finally to remove from the statute the failed social policy of the Poor Law Act with its associated harsh and utilitarian policies. The principal systems of provision were to include health, education, housing, social security and welfare benefits (see also Box 3.1).

The idea of a welfare state invokes a range of attitudes. From a collective or socialist point of view it denotes a laudable stage in the development of a state's social policy. At the other end of the spectrum are individualists from the political right, who oppose many forms of state intervention, and who interpret the welfare state as a further example of Britain's transformation into a nanny state, in which individuals have become dependent on hand-outs. There is, however, a consensus of political opinion that agrees the welfare state reflects a range of developed activities by the state which are directed towards the promotion of well-being and the protection

---

Box 3.1 Legislation for a welfare state

The programme of legislation that effectively constituted the welfare state was:

- The Education Act (1944)
- The Family Allowance Act (1945)
- The National Health Service Act (1946)
- The National Assistance Act (1948)
- The Children's Act (1948)
- The Housing Act (1949)

---

of its citizens against the rigours of the market. The term welfare state has gradually come to be associated with both the actual social welfare provision and the idea that the state itself should be the sole provider of welfare.

Activities

- In your library carry out a word search on the term welfare state.
- With your colleagues discuss some of the positive and negative connotations of the term.

The Beveridge Report

Although classed as a liberal, Beveridge was perceived by his peers as a reluctant collectivist. Beveridge's views on a publicly-funded health system originated from the ranks of the Labour Party. Beveridge believed that the spending of public money on ill-health and other social issues should be construed as an investment to facilitate a healthier workforce that would be able to promote productivity. More importantly, he argued that government control was the most efficient and cost-effective way of providing health, education, social care and other services. At the same time, Beveridge interpreted his reconstruction of public services as a means of preserving capitalism and to ward off any threat from the extreme left.

The Beveridge plan

The system of social security devised by the Beveridge committee aimed to eliminate, or at least reduce, the effects of what became known as the five giants: Want, Ignorance, Idleness, Squalor and Disease (Box 3.2). The attack on disease was based on a service structure which was to be known as the National Health Service (NHS). In Beveridge's view a comprehensive health service meant that medical treatment would be available to everyone, both in the home as well as the hospital setting.

The important period in the evolution of the

Box 3.2 The Beveridge Report

The Beveridge Report aimed to eliminate the five giants:

- Want
- Ignorance
- Idleness
- Squalor
- Disease

welfare state was between 1945 and 1948. It was during this time that Beveridge's concepts (national insurance system, universal family allowance, education reform, council housing building programme and the eventual creation of the NHS; see also Box 3.1) began to be delivered and made substantive inroads in relieving the problems of the five giants (Fraser 1984, Caul & Herron 1992, Webster 1988).

Activities

- Borrow from your library: Nicolas Timmins (1996) *The five giants: a biography of the welfare state*, and read the early chapters covering the five giants.
- Consider whether or not other issues should have been addressed, for example women's issues or services for ethnic groups.

Financial support

Beveridge's main objective was the elimination of want or poverty, which he considered to be the most important of the five giants. In this he was principally concerned with the worst excesses of the day. He was not trying to discard the forces of the market but merely put in place a strategy for correcting it as a minimal intervention to avoid unnecessary misery. Beveridge did not consider it to be his remit, nor indeed was it his intention, to make any dramatic impact on inequality or class differences and the NHS was designed on the same lines (Barry 1990, Foot 1975).

To realise this objective, his report suggested two parallel courses of action. First the govern-

ment had to pursue policies that nurtured rapid economic development and growth alongside high levels of productivity. The second was to plan for the prevention and alleviation of individual poverty resulting from those hazards or unfortunate events over which individuals have little or no control (including ill-health and seasonal or continuous unemployment). To this end his report encompassed a comprehensive scheme of social insurance which would provide financial support in any circumstances where earnings were interrupted. This would be further supplemented by the introduction of universal family allowance which would be available for children up to the age of 15 and, if in full-time education, up to 16 years of age (Rimmer et al 1981).

National Assistance and Welfare Services

The National Assistance Act was another measure that was introduced to tackle the problem of want. It stimulated the introduction of residential and community provision for the elderly, the disabled, the homeless and many other groups as an alternative to the institutional poor law workhouses. The Welfare Services Act (1949) came into operation on 1 February 1949 and further extended the function of welfare authorities, except in so far as it related to children. For this specific service separate legislation was provided.

The welfare state (and its associated legislation) was underpinned by new ideas of compassion and caring and an acceptance that some situations were beyond the control of the individual. If the welfare state was to be successful it was essential that state interventions should meet certain criteria. They must ensure that:

- basic needs were met during critical periods (unemployment, sickness or death of a spouse)
- the community should share equitably the responsibility for the provision of services
- services would be provided within a positive atmosphere and free from any form of stigma or social labelling.

Box 3.3 The principles of the Beveridge Report

The principles of the Beveridge Report can be classified under three headings.

- **Insurance**. Contributions would be universal and compulsory. In return the government would guarantee government protection, prevention, relief and compensation against loss arising out of unemployment or ill-health.
- **Payments**. Social security benefits would be at the same flat rate for all, that is subsistence level. There would be no disincentive to working.
- **Personal thrift**. Unemployment benefits should not discourage voluntary savings when people are working. Thereby re-affirmed the important position of the individual as well as government when off-setting the effects of unemployment (Marshall 1967).

Box 3.4 Social insurance

Beveridge's social insurance scheme had two components:

- A contributory insurance through which benefits could be earned through compulsory salary deductions and received during times of need or hardship.
- An assistance scheme which was non-contributory. The assistance scheme was designed to be used as a last resort or safety net to prevent hardship for those not qualifying for social insurance benefits. Benefits in these circumstances were, however, means tested.

Insurance

Insurance was the key to the success of the Beveridge Report as an alternative to taxation (Box 3.3 and Box 3.4). Contributory insurance was preferable because it explicitly linked contributions with benefits. The final package was comprehensive because people were now insured either through their own contributions, assisted contributions or, in the case of married women, benefits were paid on the basis of husbands' contributions. There were also additional benefit options for people with dependants (Williams 1990).

Activities

- List the principles upon which the welfare state was based.
- Organise a debate with your colleagues to discuss which, if any, of the services could have been provided by arrangements other than government intervention and responsibility, giving sound reasons for your answer.

THE NHS

The introduction of the NHS in 1948 is correctly described as a post-war government policy. This is not to say, however, that the government

was its sole creator, and many people assisted in the process. In October 1919 the Department of Health invited Lord Dawson of Penn to chair a committee that was given a remit to consider alternative schemes of health care which could be used for any given geographical area or community (Box 3.5). This committee quickly produced an interim report containing seminal ideas that in many respects formed the bedrock for the future NHS (Pater 1981).

Box 3.5 Principles of the Dawson Report (Dawson 1920)

- The committee recommended that the fundamental need of any community was an effective domiciliary service including the provision of general practitioners, health visitors, midwives, pharmacists and dentists.
- They agreed that institutional services should remain, as they were considered to be the most efficient modus operandi for the provision of their specialist services (i.e. mental health, tuberculosis sanitoria, care of the frail elderly).
- The committee also recommended that domiciliary services, particularly general practitioners, should place a greater emphasis on preventive medicine as well as their traditional curative function.
- They were insistent that any proposed new service should be universally available although at this stage they did not go as far as recommending that it should be free at the point of use.
- The report provided an outline idea for the provision of health centres, although they were more in line with the latter day concept of community hospitals. Dawson centres included in-patient provision and clinics where consultants could provide out-patient services (Dawson 1920).

Box 3.6 Pre-war hospital provision

Hospitals were classified under various heading and managerial arrangements, including:

- Voluntary hospitals: included the large teaching hospitals, which contained over 500 beds, in the major conurbations.
- Cottage hospitals: they were smaller in size and were distributed in medium sized towns. For the most part these hospitals provided short term medical and surgical services.
- Municipal or local authority hospitals: these emerged from the poor law workhouses. These hospitals provided acute services as well as the larger institutional services for people with learning difficulties, mental illness and infectious diseases (Chapter 2).

Wartime provision

Preparation for war

The first flickering of a new form of health care provision began around 1938. In response to an increase in the public need and, more important, the imminence of war, a group of civil servants undertook a survey of all existing municipal and voluntary hospitals. Huge inadequacies and unmet need were revealed, particularly in terms of the range of services and spread of provision (Box 3.6).

Activity

Describe briefly why the Second World War was an important influencing factor for the reorganisation of the health service.

Emergency Medical Service

Help or medical assistance of any kind during episodes of sickness could not be guaranteed and the opportunity to receive care varied considerably according to the nature of the disease, extent of personal or occupational insurance and the geographical place of residence. It was agreed by the cabinet that an acceptable standard of national health care had to be achieved. As a response, in 1939 an Emergency Medical Service was set in place. The EMS was given the responsibility of reorganising the existing system of health care into a service that could adequately respond to the demands of a war situation. The first decision made by the EMS was the creation of 12 new regions. Within each of these regions hospitals were grouped by function: emergency clearing hospitals in towns and cities; and treatment and convalescent units in the rural areas. The EMS also instituted an early form of national laboratory and blood transfusion service.

When war was declared in September 1939 treatment was provided in a limited way to military and civilian casualties free of charge. As the war progressed, however, free treatment was extended to include all workers and evacuees. Finally by the height of the conflict the list of personnel able to use this service became so extensive it included virtually the whole population. The EMS was a cornerstone in health policy because it demonstrated that, at least in the short term, it was possible to provide a comprehensive service free at the point of use. This service did not offer any ideas as to how a health care service could in the longer term be funded on a continual basis (Baggott 1994).

The road to the NHS

In 1941 the Ministry of Health announced that 'the objective of government is that, as soon as possible, after the war there should be a comprehensive hospital service available for all'. In March 1943, Ernest Brown, then Minister for Health, introduced proposals for a unified health care system with a central government department responsible for the service. The department would be advised by a council and the administration of the service would be through a system of large local government areas formed either through the existing EMS regional structure or joint authorities.

This early proposal also entailed the taking of all existing hospitals into partial national ownership and required general practitioners to become salaried employees rather than continuing as quasi-independent businesses which they had been hitherto.

Discontent

This latter proposal caused a degree of unease within the medical profession and the British Medical Association (BMA), withdrew from the negotiations, causing a temporary suspension of discussions. However, negotiations began again later in the same year after the minister said that he was prepared to concede to the medical profession a separate organisational tier for general practitioners, dentists and pharmacists, which would become known as Family Practitioner Services. This meant that GPs and the other allied professions would not be compelled to sign up to any new arrangements, although it was expected that they would.

Activities

- Discuss with your colleagues why the medical profession was particularly unhappy with the proposed reorganisation of the health service.
- List five social groups who were set to benefit directly from the changes in health care.

Amendments

By the time the White Paper was ready to be published in 1944 (Box 3.7) further important changes had been made to the benefit of the medical profession. These later amendments also ensured that the control of resources remained firmly with the large teaching hospitals. It was agreed that there would be:

- a larger medical representation on the proposed central and local bodies
- the Central Medical Board's power to control the geographical distribution of GPs was significantly diluted
- proposed Dawson-style health centres would be introduced on an experimental basis only
- the most important concession was the designation of the larger area authorities as planning bodies only.

Box 3.7 The original NHS White Paper (1944)

The radical ideas that had formed part of the Beveridge Report's proposal for a national health service were barely visible in the original White Paper published in 1944. The main proposals were:

- Planning for hospital services was to be in the hands of joint boards. These boards were to be organised on a committee system representing the constituent local authorities in the larger areas.
- Joint hospitals would be able to secure services from municipal hospitals in their own areas. Specific contracts would have covered arrangements for the purchase of services from voluntary hospitals and, if necessary, the joint board would also be able to contract for additional services from hospitals outside its own area.
- Payment for services would have come from a mixture of funds from both local and central government.
- General practitioners in local authority health centres were to be salaried and subject to greater local authority control than those who continued to operate from individual practices. Those who chose to remain outside of the new service would still be in contract with the central medical board.
- New general practitioners were restricted from setting up new practices in areas which were adjudged to have a sufficient number of doctors.

The NHS Act

The momentum for the NHS was well under way before the arrival of Aneurin Bevan in the post-war Labour government. Nevertheless, it was his personal contribution that finally spearheaded the political settlement for a service that, in spite of many flaws, was set to last virtually unaltered for nearly 30 years.

When considering a blueprint for the National Health Service, Bevan is said to have drawn from his own personal experiences of a local medical aid society. In the small village in Wales where he grew up each family was expected to contribute 3 pence for every pound that they had earned. For this contribution each family member was entitled to receive free medical and dental care, false teeth and artificial limbs, free transportation to hospital and up to 1 year's sick pay. The scheme was sufficiently comprehensive to be able to support the whole community, including the unemployed and the elderly (Honigsbaum 1989, Cassidy 1995).

Paternalist

Bevan's public image as a radical socialist and his well documented arguments with the medical profession belied a strong sense of paternalism in his political decision making. Bevan took the view that the medical profession were the experts on health matters and should therefore be listened to, even to the exclusion of others. It was this view that guaranteed for the medical profession a privileged place in any proposed new administration (Ranade 1994).

The successful implementation of the NHS was in no small measure due to Bevan's personal political skills. He has been described as a charismatic individual who enjoyed a wide circle of friends, many of whom had little in common with him politically. This characteristic enabled him to negotiate and agree separate deals with different groups within the medical profession in order to achieve consensus. Bevan realised that GPs could not be brought into the NHS without first reaching a settlement with the more politically powerful hospital consultants. This he achieved through a separate package of merit awards and attractive salary scales. Having created a degree of division within the profession, all opposition orchestrated by the BMA collapsed in spite of continuous encouragement at every stage by the opposition Conservative Party (Owen 1988).

Activities

Discuss with your colleagues:

- What is meant, in social policy terms, by the word paternalism?
- When discussing the introduction of the NHS why is it important to consider the influencing role of Aneurin Bevan?

Re-negotiating the NHS Act

As the new Minister of Health Aneurin Bevan declared that all previous negotiations were not tablets of stone and announced that he was going to re-visit the original White Paper.

The first objective for the new health service, according to the minister, was that it must be free at the point of use and divorced from an individual's ability to pay. Having removed this financial barrier, the way was then open towards achieving his other objectives for the service, which included: equity in access to health care, thereby ensuring that the only criterion for treatment was a need for care; and a universal service available to everybody in Britain irrespective of their place of domicile (Collins & Klein 1980, O'Donnell & Propper 1989).

Bevan eventually produced a scheme which differed in a number of important ways from the 1944 White Paper. The role of local authorities in hospital services was completely removed. In so doing the earlier idea of a local authority-controlled NHS had been jettisoned. He reversed many of the negotiated concessions that had previously been made to general practitioners. He did, however, concede to the medical profession the retention of: pay beds in NHS hospitals, generous rewards for hospital consultants and a large degree of medical representation on all NHS bodies.

THE NEW SERVICE

In practice the nature of services for patients did not radically alter after the introduction of the NHS on 5 July 1948. Although the ownership of assets and the source of revenue and capital changed, the culture of the institution was preserved. The principles of choice and freedom to choose remained in that individuals were still able to go to a doctor outside of the new service.

The professional autonomy of the doctor in terms of clinical judgement remained as before and doctors were also equally free to continue with private practices, even though they were contracted to working within the new service. Freedom of practice was, however, limited to doctors and allied professions. The remainder of the professional and other service staff who transferred to the NHS automatically became full-time salaried employees of what was to become the largest employer in the United Kingdom.

Box 3.8 Pressures on the NHS

The new service came under immense strain as it began to address the backlog of unmet need for medical attention. For millions of women, children, unemployed and others the NHS offered almost immediate treatment without means test, weekly stamp or prior enrolment on a medical panel:

- the NHS had cost £402 million compared to an estimated £180 million
- by the end of the first year 18 000 GPs had signed up to the new arrangements and had written 18.7 million prescriptions; 8.5 million patients had received free dental treatment; and 5.2 million people had been prescribed spectacles (Lister 1988)

Box 3.9 Tripartite structure

- **General practitioners**: were organised by family practitioner committees and were funded directly from central government. They remained largely self-employed and were remunerated on a basis of capitation fees. Similar arrangements applied to the medically allied professions, including pharmacists, dentists and opticians.
- **Local government**: the previous responsibilities of county and borough councils had accumulated from the mid 1900s. These were now drastically reduced, particularly the responsibility of providing hospital services. The focus of their residual responsibilities lay in health promotion and the prevention of ill-health, which included: maternal and child welfare, health visiting, community nursing, school medical services and other public and environmental health services.
- **Hospital authorities**: the third strand of the revised service represented by far the biggest and most important change. England was divided into fourteen regions, each containing a medical school and controlled by a regional health board that reported directly to the minister of health.

Box 3.10 Relationships with health authorities

Health authorities had a discrete relationship with two other bodies:

- community health councils, which were responsible for representing the views of consumers or patients
- local authorities, who continued with their responsibility of providing personal social services, education and housing

---

At a philosophical level there was a more obvious change in the relationship between the citizen and the state. For the first time the government had enshrined through parliament a firm and legislative commitment of state responsibility to improve the health of the nation through a comprehensive health care service (see also Box 3.8).

Organisational arrangements

The tripartite structure

The organisational form of the newly created NHS was tripartite in structure which represented a political compromise between the Labour government and the various provider groups, particularly the powerful medical profession. The components of the structure were general practitioners, local authorities and the hospital service (Box 3.9).

Regional health boards/teaching hospitals

Apart from about 200 small nursing homes or religious hospitals which were permitted to remain exempt from the national programme, all hospitals in Britain were nationalised and grouped into 377 new hospital management committees that were accountable to regional health boards (see also Box 3.10). The reason for this extensive nationalisation programme was for the most part managerial. It was believed that this policy allowed for greater organisation and

rational planning of services, thereby ensuring, even during this period, that actual need was met. In an ingenious compromise agreed between the minister and the medical profession, the major voluntary hospitals which were also centres of excellence in terms of research and medical training were exempt from this structure and granted 'teaching hospital status'. Teaching hospitals were, however, instructed to work in partnership with regional authorities and local boards, even though they were administered separately by boards of governors, who were responsible directly to the Ministry of Health.

It is probably fair to suggest that the medical profession was over-represented in both health boards and on teaching hospital committees.

Nevertheless, Bevan was adamant that the appointees for either of these managerial tiers should be based on an individual's ability and not in a representative capacity. In an open letter, he said that 'bodies shall consist of members appointed for individual suitability and experience and not as representatives or delegates of particular and possibly conflicting interests. This means that members could not be appointed to represent health workers' (cited in Klein 1983).

Activities

- List five major changes in health care that resulted from the introduction of the NHS.
- Discuss with your colleagues the principles upon which the early NHS was designed and consider whether or not the early service adhered to them.

Structural problems

From the outset the NHS was criticised for not being able to avail itself of every opportunity to promote health at both community and individual levels. It was intended that local authorities would assume responsibility for implementing this strand of the service. This, however, failed to materialise. The reasons emanated from the tripartite structure (hospital and specialist services; local health authority services; executive council for general and dental practitioners). Specifically, the problem lay in the fact that local authorities were almost completely outside of the mainstream health service. This meant that they had little involvement in the distribution of services and, more important, the allocation of central government money towards this important area (see also Box 3.11).

Additionally, because of the separation in the administrative networks, there was little communication or coordination of services between the respective bodies. The only exception to this was the vaccination and immunisation programme which in the end proved to be the most notable success of the NHS during its early years.

Box 3.11 Division of services

The division of services created an inherent weakness in the NHS and ensured:

- the continued medical dominance of hospitals and acute medicine and surgery
- an inefficient health prevention and promotion strategy
- the perpetuation of the pattern of institutional care for the elderly, mentally ill and mentally handicapped (Owen 1988)

Ill-health service

The bias of the new NHS tripartite strategy towards cure rather than prevention was further compounded by the separate planning and management of the three groups, even the administrative boundaries and funding arrangement of each sector being separate. Had the NHS taken its original form and been administered by local government, then housing and other environmental health responsibilities would have been in the same hands as the treatment services. This, it has been argued, might have created a greater stimulus for the integration of preventive and curative services. As a result issues such as the fluoridation of water supplies and a comprehensive public health education service were shelved until a later date.

Two factors heavily influenced the minister's decision to centralise and separate the structure of the service (see also Box 3.12). First, as a member of the Labour Party Bevan was ideologically committed to centralised control and second, it was argued, he was 'seduced by the claims of expertise' from the medical profession (Pater 1981).

Box 3.12 Central control

Many of the resultant criticisms of the NHS can be traced to the decision not to base services with local authorities but rather in central government control:

- the fragmentation of services into specialisations each of which contended separately for the limited available finances
- the gulf between GPs and hospital consultants (Campbell 1987)

Activities

- Consider why it was important for the government to centralise the health service.
- Discuss with your colleagues the net effect of reducing the responsibilities of local authorities.

THE POLITICS OF THE NHS

In an examination of the NHS Powell (1994) highlights the extensive parliamentary debate that preceded the implementation of the NHS Act. When the final White Paper was published, the content and philosophy were interpreted differently by members of the various political parties. To many MPs within the Labour Party the Act represented a minimum level of service upon which, through time, a more comprehensive system could eventually evolve. In the Conservative Party, on the other hand, there was a view that it represented the absolute limit of state intervention. Powell (1994) goes on to highlight the degree of confusion or misinformation that was circulating during this early period. He cites one Conservative MP as claiming that it marked the death knell of the voluntary hospital sector. At the same time a Labour MP was insisting that the Act had actually saved this form of hospital service from disappearing.

Conflicting political ideology

In spite of the early differences in interpretation, the NHS did emerge as a consensus between two different political ideologies. On the one hand pro-free-marketers within the Conservative Party who wished to retain and continue the prosperity of capitalism believed it would ward off the threat of radical socialist ideas. On the other hand, many members of the Labour Party, influenced by Fabian ideals, were satisfied that sufficient change had occurred from within, thereby offsetting any major criticisms from the far left of the party. The philosophy of the Fabians, a society formed in 1884 by the well-known philanthropists Sydney and Beatrice Webb, advocated that collective provision for

health and welfare was a necessary and inevitable development within British capitalist society (Alcock 1996).

Whether or not the NHS would have been different had Clement Attlee not achieved a landslide victory in the first post-war election is purely academic. Nevertheless the question has been pursued by Powell (1994), who contends that, for the Conservatives, the NHS Act was a high water mark of state responsibility. From this premise Powell argues that in all probability the Conservatives would have conceded greater autonomy to the voluntary hospitals as well as the medical profession. Powell goes on to suggest that, in spite of the Labour victory, the pressure from the right remained powerful enough to ensure that the eventual Act was merely a 'shell' of Labour's original intentions. To support this view Powell highlights the substantive retreats on salaries, local democracy and privilege in terms of the continued use of pay beds in the new NHS as examples of success for Conservative pressure.

Activity

With your colleagues organise a debate and examine the differences, if any, a Conservative government would have made to the NHS Act.

A unique service

The early NHS proved to be popular for the generation who grew up within the welfare state system. The creation of the National Health Service brought considerable health benefits to the general population in spite of some vigorous early opposition, particularly from the medical profession. For the first time there was a comprehensive service that was available to all and not dependent in any way on the ability of consumers to pay. It was the first health system in any Western society to offer free medical care to the entire population. Furthermore it was also the first comprehensive system to be based not on the insurance principle but on the national provision of services available, as of right, to everyone (Klein 1993).

Although regional health, district health and family practitioner authorities were almost entirely dependent on central government for finance, they did have the right and freedom to interpret national policies to suit local circumstances and needs. From this premise it can be argued that the central control of services was almost matched by an element of local autonomy. Additionally health authorities as semi-independent bodies had a reciprocal function in that they were able to exercise influence over the implementation of national decisions, which were in turn passed down to regional boards.

Parliamentary accountability

One of the peculiar aspects of the total process of creating the NHS was the relative unimportance of parliament. Uniquely, most of the debate and pressure for change emanated from extra-parliamentary forces, most specifically those organisations with a vested interest in any new form of health service. Issues were resolved and bargains were struck either without or with only token reference to parliament. The legislation that eventually appeared was, Ham (1988) contends, little more than a record of the decisions that had been made. Paradoxically, once the legislation had been enshrined, with the health service becoming the direct responsibility of the Minister of Health, the inverse happened. All decisions from the date of the commencement of the NHS became the subject of heated political debate and health care policy became and remains an essential component of any potential government's election manifesto.

The fact that the Secretary of State for Health and Social Services was accountable to parliament was a phenomenon unique to Britain and does not occur in other national health care systems. The existence of parliamentary accountability, through the minister, in many ways acted as a centralising influence. It ensured that the secretary of state had a significant role and input in the planning and organising of services. Conversely, it also ensured that health care

became a perennial political issue, which at different times both influenced and inhibited decision making and any potential for change (Ham 1988).

Funding problems

Many of the major funding problems that beset the NHS following the first 6 years of its inception can be attributed to the confusing and medically-orientated managerial arrangements. However, it must also be remembered that the pre-existing infrastructure also added to the difficulties of ensuring a fair distribution of services. Many of the hospitals that the new NHS inherited had been built in the 19th century and were totally unsuited to the rapidly changing and increasingly technological health service that emerged.

Given the fact that this was a post-war period and the treasury was attempting to restore some solidity to the economic order, it was impossible for the government to release any capital spending money. As a result it was the 1960s before any new hospitals were erected.

When Bevan introduced the NHS the degree of central control via the Ministry of Health was maximised. He considered that this was the best and fairest way of ensuring an equal distribution throughout the length and breadth of the country, a policy that dated back to the Poor Law Relief Act (1834). Although a degree of balance between this centralised control and the autonomy of local authorities to provide discrete and different services has evolved, the original idea of a nationally similar structure and service did persist. In an interview with future staff of the NHS Bevan honestly admitted that 'we will never have all we need ... This service must always be changing, growing and improving, it must always appear inadequate' (Foot 1975).

 Activity

Consider the reasons why funding for health care was a particular issue during the early years of the NHS.

Public or private services

The programme of social legislation that constituted the welfare state and the NHS has been described as evolutionary rather than revolutionary. It was evolutionary in the sense that it built on pre-existing legislation and was not revolutionary because there was no consistent underlying philosophy of welfarism (Barry 1990, Jones 1992). Many of the new arrangements have been described as haphazard and not developed from a rational plan but simply reactions to particular circumstances (namely the five giants: want, ignorance, idleness, squalor and disease).

Additionally, the social or collective model of providing health care has not been without its critics, principally because in the longer term the model has to some extent not matched its high ideals. Many subsequent studies have revealed that the better off have continued to have better access to services and have also been able to make better use of them (Black Report 1979, Titmuss 1974, 1979).

With the exception of income maintenance for the poor, which can be justified in terms of public good, the major services associated with the welfare state (education, health care, pensions) could, it has been argued, have quite easily been provided by and referred to as private services. This view, however, was not publicly popular because the concept of socialised medicine does form the cutting edge in the clash of interests between the rich and poor (Graham 1990).

Conclusion

Beveridge and his committee dominated health and social services in the 1940s. The steps undertaken during this period were described as bold, creative and compassionate. Health was interpreted as an investment rather than a consumption or a drain on resources, and this view remained virtually unchallenged until the NHS became operational. It was only when the costs of sustaining the service began to spiral that serious questions were posed. As a result the much heralded comprehensive service for all was described as over-optimistic and accusations were made that the early pioneers had not properly considered the potential pitfalls.

When the NHS was introduced it was hoped that the demand for service would not exceed the ability of the government to provide or, more appropriately, pay for. This view originated with the Beveridge Report which predicted that once the 'pool of sickness' in society had been addressed and the endemic diseases suppressed, the NHS would begin to cater for a healthier population. It was also anticipated that the costs of providing a service would stabilise for at least 20 years after its introduction. This belief was based on the assumption that the demand for services was finite and that if financial resources could be ring-fenced to allow specific and new health care problems to be addressed and alleviated, expenditure could be self-limiting. This proved, however, not to be the case as the NHS rapidly diversified and costs increased beyond all expectation.

The medical influence during the early period of the NHS laid the foundation for the early jettisoning of the idea that the service should have an equal focus on prevention of ill-health and health education to that of its role as a curative service, reacting to the presence of disease or ill-health. This imbalance has only recently begun to be addressed in a meaningful way (Klein 1993, Klein & O'Higgins 1985).

Activities

Having read this chapter and tried some of the study exercises, work your way through the following:

- The NHS has been described as the envy of the world – with your colleagues discuss this statement.
- Discuss with your colleagues the value of the NHS in terms of reducing the 'five giants'.
- Talk to an older relative who remembers the immediate post-war period and ascertain how important the implementation of the welfare state was at the time.
- Contrast this universal policy with the harsh utilitarian ideas associated with the poor law that were discussed in Chapter 2.
- Carry out a small search of the literature on another system of health and welfare provision in a developed country (suggest France, Sweden, Holland or Germany) and compare your findings with the British system.

REFERENCES

Alcock P 1996 Social policy in Britain: themes and issues. Macmillan, London

Barry N 1990 Welfare. Open University Press, Milton Keynes

Baggott R 1994 Health and health care in Britain. Macmillan, London

Black Report 1979 Inequalities and health. Department of Health and Social Security

Campbell J 1987 Nye Bevan and the mirage of British socialism. Weidenfeld and Nicolson, London

Cassidy J 1995 From cradle to grave. Nursing Times 91(27):14–15

Caul B, Heron S 1992 A service for the people: origins and development of the personal and social services of Northern Ireland. Universities Press, Belfast

Collins E, Klein R 1980 Equity and the NHS: self-reported morbidity, access and primary care. British Medical Journal 281:1111–1115

Dawson, Lord 1920 Interim report on the future provision of medical and allied services. Cmd 693, HMSO, London

Foot M 1975 Aneurin Bevan. Paladin/Granada, London

Fraser D 1984 The evolution of the British welfare state. Macmillan, London

Graham G 1990 Contemporary social philosophy. Blackwell, Oxford

Ham C 1988 Health policy in Britain, 2nd edn. Macmillan, London

Honigsbaum F 1989 Health, happiness and security: the creation of the National Health Service. Routledge, London

Jones K 1991 The making of social policy in Britain, 1830–1990. Athlone Press, London

Klein R, O'Higgins M (eds) 1985 The future of welfare. Blackwell, Oxford

Klein R 1993 Dimensions of rationing: who should do what. British Medical Journal 307:309–311

Klein R 1983 The politics of the National Health Service. Longman, Harlow

Lister J 1988 Cutting the lifeline: the fight for the NHS. Journeyman, London

Marshall H 1967 Social policy in the twentieth century. Hutchinson, London

O'Donnell O, Propper C 1989 Equity and the distribution of NHS resources. (Welfare State Discussion Paper WSP/45.) London School of Economics, London

Owen D 1988 Our NHS. Pan, London

Pater J 1981 The making of the National Health Service. King Edward's Hospital Fund, London

Powell 1994 The forgotten anniversary? An examination of the 1944 White Paper, 'A National Health Service'. Social Policy and Administration 28(4):333–343

Ranade W 1994 A future for the NHS? Health care in the 1990s. Longman, London

Rimmer L, Allsop J, Gaffin J, Robinson K 1981 The nurse and the welfare state. H M and M, London

Timmins N 1995 The five giants: a biography of the welfare state. Fontana Press, London

Titmuss R 1974 Essays on the welfare state. Unwin, London

Titmuss R 1979 Commitment to welfare. Allen and Unwin, London

Webster C 1988 The health services since the war, volume 1. HMSO, London

Williams F 1990 Social policy: a critical introduction. Polity Press, Cambridge

4

The process of policy implementation

Fred Sutton

At the end of the chapter the student will be able to:

- **understand the aims and constraints on social policy**
- **understand how policies can be affected**
- **understand how policies are implemented in the UK**

Introduction

For policies to come into being there must first be a perceived social problem. However, the existence of a problem is not sufficient to guarantee that policy will be implemented (or changed) to affect the problem. Along with the existence of the problem there must also be the means to draw attention to it. This can come about, for example, through the actions of pressure groups, or through media attention. Even when these conditions are met there may be a perceived change in policy or perhaps a change in the emphasis of a policy, but this may be just a token gesture. If, for example, insufficient resources are set aside for the implementation of the policy then any changes made may have no effect (Hall 1975). This chapter will discuss some of the influences on social and health policies and how they are formulated and implemented in the UK.

INFLUENTIAL GROUPS

Pressure groups

Pressure groups can make demands on a wide

range of issues. The success of pressure groups can depend on a number of elements. Their relationship with those making policy can be a crucial factor. If a minister has a 'pet' project, then she may welcome the advances of pressure groups, if it will strengthen her hand in funding negotiations with the Treasury.

If pressure groups are unsuccessful in trying to affect government policy, then they can turn to parliament and the media. They can get MPs who are sympathetic to their cause to raise questions in the House of Commons, or bring forward a private member's bill, such as David Alton's Abortion Bill, which reduced the gestation time limit for abortions from 28 to 24 weeks. Although the pressure group may not achieve exactly what they started out to, there may well be a compromise which will affect policy. Along with this they can approach the media to see if they will take up their cause. In recent years the media can be seen to have had an important effect in a number of ways. Newspaper campaigns can call for changes to policy, or highlight specific problem areas. Documentaries on television can also bring problems to the fore. In an age where political parties are becoming more sensitive to media attention, this can have important ramifications.

Activities

- Form a list of pressure groups.
- Discuss with your teacher how they are able to influence policy decisions.

Ministers and civil servants

Other ways in which policy can be changed is from ministers and civil servants. A new secretary of state is liable to have ideas that she would like to implement. This can happen specifically with a new government who may have ideas, formulated whilst in opposition, which may be in direct contrast to prevailing policy. For example, the change in government in 1979 brought a change in philosophy, a move towards the introduction of privatised industries and the free market, along with the growth of the private health sector.

Although ministers and governments will change, civil servants remain in position. This can lead to a continuity with policy, they may also have their own ideas on policy. This may lead to a more conservative approach to policy formation as they will have to deal with the pressure groups once the ministers have moved on. They may not necessarily pursue their own policies against the ministers' preferences, but they may attempt to temper more controversial aspects of the policy.

Private sector influence

Industry can also have an effect on policy implementation, specifically in health policy. Private providers may attempt to influence policy makers, as the private sector has an interest in the policies that the government pursues. Another influence from the private sector is those that supply the NHS with equipment, the drug industry and those firms that are trying for contracts to supply services, such as cleaning. Other industries have an interest in goods which are deemed to be harmful to health, such as alcohol and tobacco. These industries are relatively free from regulation restrictions despite the negative medical evidence.

There is an assumption that if a large number of people all make individual decisions then the extremes are likely to cancel each other out, and the decisions made will tend towards the benefit of society as a whole. In some ways this is looking at how the 'average' member of society will react. This approach assumes that everyone has the ability to take part in the decisions that are made. In reality policies are decided by the government, and so decisions will be taken by MPs who are either representing the constituents who voted for them, or following party dogma. They may well ignore minorities, whose views are very important in terms of social policy (Ham 1992).

Activity

Discuss with your colleagues why the private sector is an important consideration in social policy.

PARLIAMENT

After a general election the leader with the largest single party in the House of Commons forms a government and the leader becomes the prime minister. The PM then appoints about 100 ministers, from among whom the cabinet is selected. Ministers are responsible for the day-to-day running of the government's business through the major departments of state. These include the Treasury, which is responsible for all matters to do with finance, and the Department of Health. Most of the work is carried out by civil servants, although ministers are still held responsible for the work done. Parliament also monitors the work of government departments through a system of select committees. The idea behind parliament is that it is there to pass legislation, examine public expenditure and control the government. In practice its power to carry out these functions is limited. As long as there is a government majority, then parliament effectively has few significant powers.

The task of securing the government majority in the House of Commons falls to the party whips. They ensure that MPs are present to vote, and the government legislative programme is passed. Most legislation originates from the government, and bills have to go through a number of stages before becoming law. Parliamentary debates on legislation provide an opportunity for party views to be reiterated, and occasionally the government will accept amendments put forward by the opposition parties. On occasions, important legislation may be defeated or withdrawn, but the existence of a parliamentary majority coupled with strong party discipline ensures that these occasions will be rare (Ham 1992).

Individual MPs are able to use parliament in two other main ways. First they can put down parliamentary questions, asking ministers about aspects of their work for which they are responsible. Some of these questions receive written replies, while others are oral, where they can then ask another question. MPs can also raise adjournment debates, which are usually on local or constituency issues.

Activities

- Organise your class into a number of different groups and arrange seminars to discuss the legislation process for:
  — England and Wales
  — Scotland
  — Northern Ireland.
- Discuss the similarities and differences.

Select committees

Recently there has been the use of select committees, which are made up of MPs who investigate particular subjects and publish reports on their findings. Although they were established in response to the decline in the power of the Commons to control the government, their impact is limited. They are effective only if the government is willing to accept their recommendations. Although it is expected that departments will respond to committee reports, this does not mean that the committee findings will have any influence on policy. There is an idea that select committees are useful for gauging public reaction to the policy recommendations. If there is a very unfavourable reaction to the announcement of select committee findings, then the government may take note of the outcry before it decides on its 'preferred' policy.

LOCAL GOVERNMENT

The major policy decisions are taken centrally, with routine administrative decisions taken by locally-based civil servants. For example the local DSS offices administer the benefit system, while they are employed centrally. Along with this, all countries of a significant size decentralise some of the basic tasks of governance towards local authorities. Policy making responsibilities in a number of service provision areas is handed to locally-elected regional government. Local authorities decide on the provision of local services in accordance with the wishes and needs of the residents of the locality. In the UK, local government does not necessarily mean self-government. Local authorities can do only what they are statutorily permitted to do. If a local authority does something it is not allowed to do, or spends money that it is not statutorily authorised to spend, it will be deemed to have acted beyond its power, and therefore illegally. For example in the 1980s Derek Hatton and the Labour-run Liverpool Council were suspended for bankrupting the local authority.

The main characteristic of local authorities, which sets them apart from other regional bodies, is that they are directly elected. They are not composed of civil servants, or government appointees, but consist of local people chosen by local people to represent their interests. A further distinction is that local authorities have the power to tax local residents to raise revenue, although most local government funds come directly from central government (Wilson & Game 1994).

Although they are locally elected, the government retains the power to suspend and abolish local councils. One of the problems from the point of view of central government is the possible refusal of local authorities to carry out the government's wishes. This can happen when the local authority is governed by members of the opposition party, who may try to go against the government's wishes. The Conservative government, from 1979 onwards, regarded local government as wasteful, irresponsible and out of control. With this in mind they produced a large amount of legislation aimed at remodelling them. They abolished the Greater London Council and the six metropolitan county councils, scaled down local education authorities, removing their responsibility for polytechnics, further education and sixth form colleges, school budgets and opted out schools. They introduced competitive tendering for services such as refuse

collection, cleaning, catering and so on, which now tend to be contracted out to the private sector. Some service responsibilities have been removed from local authority control and given to government appointed agencies, such as the Urban Development Corporations for inner city development, Training and Enterprise Councils and Housing Action Trusts. So there has been a growth in non-elected local government. Along with this, the local taxation system has undergone a series of reforms. Government ministers are now able to cap the councils' levels of spending, and limit the amount of tax they can raise, and so can now to some extent control their budgets.

Personal social services come under the control of local authorities. The relevant authorities are county councils in shire areas and borough councils in metropolitan areas. Local elections give local authorities an independent power base, while the existence of the council tax as a source of revenue provides the means by which the authorities can determine spending levels. In practice central government involvement in local affairs has increased in recent years, but local authorities retain some freedom to decide on the quality of services to be provided in their areas. With the government increasing the use of grant capping, decisions on quality of services are becoming more difficult, as to improve or maintain the quality of one service may result in the decline of another. As would be expected, local autonomy also means local variation, and there are wide differences in spending levels and types of services provided.

Activities

- Discuss ways in which you would attempt to influence government policy.
- How could you raise public awareness?

Health policy responsibilities

The Secretary of State for Health has overall responsibility for providing health services, which it discharges through NHS authorities who are their agents. Special Health Authorities, National Health Service Trusts and Family Health Services Authorities administer services at local level, but these authorities do not simply carry out the secretary of state's wishes. NHS authorities have important policy-making responsibilities in their own right, and they interpret national policies to suit local circumstances. On the other hand, unlike local authorities, they lack the legitimacy derived from elections and have no significant independent sources of revenue.

Health policy is not determined by ministers alone; the medical profession is also involved in the management of health services at several different points. Within the Department of Health and through the department's consultative machinery, professions contribute to policy making. Family Health Services Authorities include a GP among their membership and receive advice from local medical committees. Under the NHS reforms they have also started appointing independent medical advisers. Also, NHS trusts usually include a medical director on their boards and rely extensively on advice received from their medical staff.

Quangos

There has been a transformation in the way that local communities have been governed. In the past local authorities were the leaders of the community. They now have to share powers with appointed bodies known as quangos (short for quasi-autonomous non-governmental organisations). Many of the functions of local authorities have been removed. Britain's city-wide authorities have been abolished; involvement of councils in higher education and training has been all but terminated; and councils have had to privatise services like refuse collection.

The aim behind the changes in the provision of services is to empower consumers; for example the opting out of schools from local authorities is supposed to hand power to parents. However, this has not necessarily happened in practice, either in education or in the provision of other services. One of the main problems with quangos

is that the people involved tend to be appointed by government ministers. Public Bodies 1993, a publication from the Cabinet Office, says that ministers are responsible for 42 600 appointments to public bodies. In any one year ministers make or renew about 10 000 of them. In written answers to parliamentary questions the government has revealed that in 1992 it advertised only 24 of these appointments (Wilson 1994).

Local accountability

Local authorities are accountable to the public, mainly through the fact that they are elected bodies, and can be removed from power at the next local election. Quangos are not elected bodies, and there are several other differences between quangos and local authorities (Box 4.1). Most local quangos are subject to fewer checks and controls than local authorities. Local councils, unlike quangos, are obliged to publish auditors' criticisms. Every local authority has an accounting officer who is responsible for checking that funds are properly spent, but some quangos do not. Councillors are liable to be surcharged for the improper use of public funds; quango board members are not. Local authorities have to keep a register of councillors' interests; quangos keep no such list for their board members. Council meetings are open to the public, but of all the quangos, only the health authorities are required to admit the public. Many quangos have no code of conduct to promote a public service ethos. Most quango board members have little contact with the people on whose behalf

---

Box 4.1 Quangos

Key differences between a quango and a public service are that in quangos:

- Members are appointed not elected
- There is no requirement to publish auditor's review
- There is no requirement to declare member's private interests
- There is no requirement for open and public meetings
- Quangos have limited contact with the service that is provided

they administer services, whereas many councillors regard it as their duty to help an elector with a problem. Councillors hold regular surgeries and may receive huge postbags.

In 1986 the Widdicombe inquiry into local government found that a third of those surveyed knew who one of their councillors was, while 20% had had contact with a councillor. At the moment quangos face few of the statutory obligations that apply to local authorities, such as public access to their meetings. In written evidence to the Nolan Committee on Standards in Public Life (1995), the minister for public service, David Hunt, said such statutory controls were not needed as quangos were responsible to ministers, who would apply any necessary discipline. Nor was he concerned that neither the National Audit Office nor the Audit Commission can investigate some quangos, such as the scandal-prone training and enterprise councils.

OPENNESS

In April 1994 the government introduced a code of practice governing access to official information in response to criticisms of secrecy. The code's arbiter was the Parliamentary Commissioner for Administration, who is known as the ombudsman. The predicted move to openness from the introduction of the code has not materialised for a number of reasons. Many parts of government business are exempt from disclosure, including any information which would 'harm the frankness and candour of internal discussion'. This includes not only proceedings of cabinet and cabinet committees, but also the factual reports on which the advice is based. It also covers communications between departments and public bodies, including independent industry regulators, and thousands of quangos, as well as between public officials and private firms. Another problem is that rather than complain to the ombudsman directly, people must go through an MP. Before the ombudsman will consider a complaint, the department which has refused a request for information has to be given the opportunity to review its decision. These requests for information should be

answered within 20 days, but some departments have multi-layered internal review procedures which delay matters for months. Additionally the code commits departments to supplying only a summary of the information, not the actual documents, so it is difficult to know to what extent these extracts of official documents have been edited. Without statutory backing, access to official information remains at the whim of ministers. They can deny the ombudsman access to the documents he needs to assess where the public interest lies. In any case, ministers can ignore a ruling by the ombudsman and have done so on a number of occasions. If a minister is able to reject an ombudsman's findings, then it could be suggested that there is little point in having an ombudsman. Nor is there any reason why local councils should not deal with the reports of the local ombudsman in a similar fashion. If the credibility of the ombudsman is diminished, then one of the few defences the people have against administrative power is effectively removed.

THE 1979–1997 CONSERVATIVE GOVERNMENT APPROACH

In 1979 the incoming Conservative government committed itself to a monetary stance, in contrast to the traditional Keynesian policies generally pursued for the previous 30 years. This policy involved strict control of public expenditure. Their philosophy was that the market is seen as the best provider of goods and services, including forms of welfare other than the residual minimum. They encouraged people to provide for themselves by buying private insurance and private pension plans. The idea was that the state should only intervene in the market as a last resort. They wanted to reduce the role of the government in the belief that the market is most efficient when left to its own devices.

The reduction in the role of government led to the promotion of independent education and the introduction of the assisted places scheme. Coupled with this was the 'right to buy' policy for council house tenants, which led to an unprecedented increase in house ownership. Public housing that was removed from local authority control was not replaced by building new houses and so the stock of the public housing sector was reduced, thereby limiting the local authority's ability to provide council housing.

Paternalism

The change in ideology towards the free-market system was partly in response to the perceived paternalistic nature of the state, that is the view that the state knows best. In this way the state plays the role of the parent with the individual citizen playing the role of the child. So the state will look after the 'child' and will do what it considers to be in the best interests of the individual, irrespective of what that individual may desire. Continuing the analogy, the state acts in the same way as a parent would, for example preventing the child from eating sweets, even though that is what the child wants, in order to protect the child's teeth for the future. We have many paternalistic laws in place which are aimed at protecting the individual whilst restricting their freedom to choose, for example the wearing of seatbelts, the regulation of drugs and so on (Häyry 1991).

One of the criticisms levelled against this paternalistic approach is that it removes an individual's right to choose. This move away from the 'nanny' state is not confined to the left or the right, but is accepted by both, although there are some contradictions. The right have generally favoured a move towards the operation of free markets, whereas the left has traditionally gone for the nationalised institutions, along with a socialist basis for education and health. The right has tried to restrict what could be termed paternalistic legislation, such as a minimum working week, and a minimum wage. Yet at the same time it has tried to promote its own particular brand of morals and erode the standing of certain groups, such as single parents. Those who would be termed more liberal have championed the right of people to have more freedom, but at the same time have advocated that the state knows best in terms of education matters, for example.

Activities

List some of the functions of:

- Parliamentary select committees.
- Quangos.

THE FREE-MARKET SYSTEM

The idea behind a market system is that it brings together buyers and sellers who exchange goods at a mutually acceptable rate. The notion of efficiency within the market system focuses upon a particular type of firm, the perfectly competitive firm. If perfect competition existed in all sectors of the economy, and if distribution was socially acceptable, it can be argued that the use of society's resources would be optimised. But perfectly competitive firms have certain attributes which are not found in the real world (Taylor 1990).

The idea is that there is a number of firms who are all producing the same product, and consumers will choose between these products on the basis of quality and price. There is perceived to be free entry into the market for new firms, and so only efficient firms will survive. Those firms who are inefficient will not be able to sell their products as consumers will turn to a cheaper alternative. Consumers also have perfect knowledge of the market so they know all about what is being produced and how much it will cost. Using this information they will purchase the products which are of the best quality and at the cheapest price. This approach is unrealistic in the real world for a number of reasons. One reason is that it totally ignores the effect of advertising and branding of goods to encourage brand loyalty, one result of which is that consumers will continue to purchase certain known brands irrespective of the cheaper alternatives because of what they believe to be the extra kudos they get from purchasing that particular item. Another reason is that entry into markets can have explicit and implicit restrictions. To enter into the car industry, for example, would require huge financial backing; in many industries the existence of patents can restrict other firms from using new technology, so giving the patent owner an advantage.

A further concept in this policy was the encouragement of private provision of services in a wide range of areas of social policy. The boost to private providers of residential care by allowing residents fees to be paid by the DSS, and tax incentives to some groups taking out private health insurance, are two illustrations of what has become a comprehensive shift towards the private sector as a leading contender in the provision of welfare.

Conclusion

The pace of change in the provision of welfare intensified in the late 1980s. Services such as housing have become increasingly marginalised, whilst legislation on education has had the effect of introducing more elements of supposed consumer choice into the public sector. In the health services developments include both a greater move towards a form of market system within the health service, and greater incentives for individuals to switch to private health care as an alternative to the NHS. Thus the third term of office for the Conservative government reinforced the concept of selective measures in welfare services and the use of the private sector wherever possible. In part the Conservative government was able to use a growing disillusionment with the welfare state amongst politicians, academics and society itself to support its changes. Systematic study of the scope and effect of social provisions has developed over the past 40 years, since the inception of the welfare state, to reveal the inequalities that still exist within the system. Thus access to education has proved to be far from equal, poverty exists despite the introduction of income support and a contributory system of benefits, and inequalities in health between the social classes remain despite the introduction of a national health service. In addition there had been growing discontent with the ways in which the services are delivered.

The income maintenance system and the health services have both been criticised for being too impersonal, too remote from the needs of those they serve, too intimidating and too bureaucratic. Consumers have voiced discontent with a variety of services (the officialdom of the housing authorities or of social services, for example), whilst those on the left have been critical of the social controls within the delivery of welfare services.

The Conservative government's commitment to restricting state services to those who demonstrate genuine need, measured by means tests, and to increasing private provision as an alternative to state services must be seen within the context of existing concern over the ability of social policy to provide for the needs of all.

Activities

- Discuss the changes in the policy process since 1979.
- Discuss any improvements or downfalls in the democratic process.
- Discuss what is meant by the terms openness and accountability in government.
- List some ways in which consecutive governments have sought to address these issues.

REFERENCES

Hall P 1975 Change, choice and conflict in social policy. Gower, Aldershot

Ham C 1992 Health policy in Britain. Macmillan, London

Häyry H 1991 The limits of medical paternalism. Routledge, London

Taylor I 1990 The social effects of free market policies. Prentice Hall/Harvester Wheatsheaf, Hemel Hempstead

Wilson D, Game C 1994 Local government in the United Kingdom. Macmillan, London

5

Social issues and health

Siân P. Thomas

At the end of this chapter the reader should be able to:

- **understand the relationship between social issues and health**
- **discuss the relationships between stratification and health with a focus on class and ethnic groups**
- **consider health chances concentrating on inequalities in health and the impact of lifestyles, behaviour, poverty and environment**
- **have an awareness of social models of health practice and of initiatives to address imbalances in relationships between different social groups and health care**

Introduction

Although there are health inequalities between individuals based on biological and genetic background, health and illness are not only determined by physical and mental conditions. Wider social influences have a profound effect on our experiences of and the occurrence of illness and disease. Inequalities can often result from comparative disadvantage between different groups of people. Social factors can either improve our health or contribute to sickness and disease. Our health is therefore the result of an elaborate interaction between our physical, mental and social states.

This chapter seeks to explore the complex relationship between social issues and health. It aims to provide readers with an introduction to some of the main forms of social difference in our society. In particular the focus will be on the disparities in health between people of different occupational status and ethnic groups. Gender, another key form of social division, is explored in detail in Chapter 6.

SOCIAL ISSUES AND HEALTH CARE: A COMPLEX RELATIONSHIP

At the creation of the National Health Service (NHS) (see Chapter 3), the intention was to provide universal health services available to all with every person receiving the same standard of service. Indeed, Aneurin Bevan, the Minister for Health, describing the NHS to the House of Commons in 1946, stated that there was to be 'no limitation on the kind of assistance given – the general practitioner service, the specialist, the hospitals, eye treatment, spectacles, dental treatment, hearing facilities, all these are to be made available free' (quoted in Webster 1991).

However, despite the optimism surrounding the beginnings of the NHS, the realities then and now suggest that health services are not experienced by all in the same way. The distribution of health resources, the different patterns of illness suffered and other contributing factors ensure that different groups within the UK have unequal health needs and experience the unequal provision of health care. It is therefore important to be able to distinguish between the ideal that services are available to all free at the point of use with the reality of vastly different experiences.

Explanations as to why these differences between social groups exist are complex. First of all, we need to have an understanding of the social factors which determine how one individual's life experiences vary from another's. Mitchell (1984, pp. 105–106) sought to explain the areas of social relations which need to be assessed:

To explore what is making us ill we have to look at the relationship between women and men, between white and black people, between employee and employer, and we have to look at the way work is organised, the hours of work, the division of labour, how caring for children, sick and very elderly people, making food and doing housework is organised, how houses are built, how cities are planned, and who decides, who is in control and where the power lies.

STRATIFICATION AND HEALTH

Class

A key phrase used to describe inequalities is social stratification. Social stratification is a way of outlining the layers of society from top to bottom. Within Western societies the basic form of stratification is based on economic difference. That is to say difference based on employment status, job type and level of income. These layers have been described as 'class' by many major theorists.

The most influential approaches to stratification in modern societies have been the theories of Karl Marx (1818–1883) and Max Weber (1864–1920). The majority of theories developed since have been indebted to the concepts of these two German theorists.

Marx

In Marx's view a class is a collection of people who have a common relationship to the means of production (The means of production being how they earn a living.) Within modern industrial societies, Marx identified two principal classes. The bourgeoisie or capitalists who are the business owners, and the proletariat or working classes who sell their labour. As a result of the division of labour and the creation of profit from industry, the relationship between the classes is exploitative as some have greater access to material resources than others.

Marx recognised that real class systems (as opposed to theoretical systems) were more complex due to transitional classes left over from previous production systems which persist alongside modern industry (e.g. peasants from agriculture-based systems). He also recognised the divisions which can exist within a class, for example between small business owners and those owning large companies within the capitalist class or between the long-term unemployed and the employed within the working class.

Weber

Max Weber developed a significant alternative to Marx's view of class. Whereas Weber accepts Marx's definition of class based on relationships to the means of production and objective economic inequalities in society, he argues that other economic differences are also important. In particular, Weber emphasises the sharing of a common market position by those with similar skills, qualifications and other marketable assets which influence the type of jobs individuals can attain.

Aside from class, Weber introduced the concepts of status and party as further aspects of stratification. Status is concerned with positive or negative criteria and common lifestyles, such as those of ethnic groups or other groupings of people, who either have high prestige or alternatively who are discriminated against. Therefore, whereas class may be seen as objective, status relies on subjective views of lifestyles. Weber's concept of party refers to groups who are bound by common backgrounds, aims or interests. A party can run across class divisions, and examples include religious or nationalist groups.

Later theories

Marx and Weber's theories of stratification are still currently utilised, but usually with some alterations. Even though it may be argued that class differences when Marx and Weber were writing were more pronounced than they are today, class differences still persist through variations in wealth and income, status and affiliation. Many subsequent theoretical approaches are heavily influenced by these theories.

Giddens (1993, p. 215) describes class as 'a large-scale grouping of people who share common economic resources, which strongly influence the types of lifestyle they are able to lead. Ownership of wealth, together with occupation, are the chief bases of class differences'. Table 5.1

Table 5.1 Class in modern Western society (after Giddens 1993)

Upper class	Those who own or directly control productive resources – the wealthy, employers, industrialists
Middle class	Most white collar employees and professionals
Working class	Blue collar and manual jobs

outlines Giddens's view of the main classes in modern Western society.

Social mobility

Class systems are fluid and the boundaries between classes not clearly established. An individual's status is not a fixed entity, as mobility can occur both up and down the layers of society. With status ascribed to particular types of work, it is possible to either move up the layers of society as a result of being employed in a different type of work, or to move down a layer, through for example unemployment. Social mobility is a term used to describe the movement of an individual or group from one position in the social structure of society to another.

Hence although your class position may be heavily influenced by that of your family, it is not predetermined at birth. A particular class is not ascribed to a person for life, but rather social mobility enables individuals to move up or down in the class structure according to individual circumstances.

Economic differences

The differentiating factor of economic difference between individuals is important, as our access to material resources and their availability to us determines a great deal about our lives, including our experience of health and illness. Access or lack of access to economic security significantly affects the quality and quantity of life.

Occupation

Common sense understandings of class often rely on a classification of occupations. The

Box 5.1 Standard occupational classification (after Office for National Statistics 1989)

This system has nine levels of occupational segregation:

- managers and administrators
- professionals
- associate professional and technical
- clerical and secretarial
- craft and skilled manual
- personal and protective services
- sales
- plant and machine operatives
- others.

Activities

- List five indicators of social status and class in British society.
- Discuss with your friends how class can impact on health.

Office for National Statistics' classification of occupations (1989) is one such method, based on the type of work done as described by job title and job description (Box 5.1). Many health care professionals, such as registered nurses, physiotherapists and occupational therapists, could be classified as associate professionals.

The application of the Registrar General's classification system has been criticised (Montgomery & Carter-Pokras 1993, Najman 1993) as contemporary modifications in occupational structure have meant that it fails to take account of all economic groups, including the unemployed. Instead a wider view of economic inequality should be utilised.

Definitions of class and occupational groupings therefore stress the importance of income and economic status. Our level of income impacts on our way of life. If affects where we live and how we live. It influences the type of housing we live in, our ability to adequately clothe ourselves and furnish our homes. It impacts on the food and drink we consume, our use of fuel and our purchase of consumer goods. It therefore controls our access to the basic elements which contribute to the quality of our life and ultimately our health.

Empirical evidence concerning class and occupational differences in contemporary Britain shows the unequal experience of health and illness. As Moore & Harrison (1995, p. 221) have summarised: 'Good health generally appears to be associated with wealth, while ill health appears to accompany poverty and social deprivation'.

POVERTY AND HEALTH CHANCES

A primary difficulty in comprehending inequalities in health is substantiating a connection between poverty and ill-health. Poverty is a difficult concept to define. A common distinction that is made is between absolute and relative definitions of poverty. Absolute poverty refers to circumstances in which a person cannot afford the amenities needed for subsistence. In contrast, relative poverty may be defined as a situation where a person lacks basic resources in comparison to the standard of living of others in the society. In other words their standard of living is comparatively worse relative to that of the average standard of living.

Relative poverty

Many contemporary writers, of whom the most influential is perhaps Townsend (1979), have contended that relative poverty is the most appropriate measure of poverty in modern Britain. Criticism of absolute poverty points to the fact that an individual may have enough to survive, but this is not necessarily equivalent to a reasonable standard of living, and indeed may result in the individual becoming marginalised from society.

A measure used by Townsend (1979) to outline relative poverty is an individual's position against social security levels. The receiving of income support and the individual's income as a percentage of average income are key measures.

Causes of poverty

Townsend (1979) outlined the following as the major causes of poverty: low pay, ill-health, loss of the breadwinner, unemployment and old age. Older people, single parents, the low paid, the long term sick and disabled, and the unemployed were identified as the key groups living in poverty. The major causes of poverty are therefore social misfortune as well as economic and structural factors.

At practically each stage in the life cycle inequalities in health have been found (Townsend et al 1992). Social difference resulting from a variety of forms of social stratification relate to our health chances throughout our life cycle. Our social situation and that of our family affects our health chances from birth through life to death. Lifestyle, the effect of social institutions, the role health services play, all interact to influence and affect our health chances.

Birth, infancy and childhood

Birth, infancy and childhood are key stages of the life cycle. Social stratification is strongly connected to an individual's chance of survival at birth and during their first 12 months. Empirical evidence (Reid 1989) shows that there are social class variations in the length of pregnancy, with women from partly skilled and unskilled groups experiencing curtailed pregnancies in comparison with those in professional groups who are more likely to experience mature pregnancies. Those in lower occupational groups are also more likely to experience higher rates of infant mortality, and are more likely to have babies with lower birth weights, which can have an effect on the subsequent development of the child.

Old age

At the other end of the life cycle, older people are the largest low income group in the UK (Teale 1996). Adequate income is an essential factor in enabling older people to have a reasonable standard of living. While those with occupational pensions may enjoy a comfortable standard of living, those without may face financial hardship. Of the 10 million people of pensionable age (currently age 60 for women and 65 for men) more than 1.5 million people

over 60 receive income support because of low income. It is also estimated that at least half a million pensioners who are eligible for income support do not claim.

Teale (1996) proposes explanations as to why older people on the whole are significantly worse off than the remaining population:

- The basic state pension was 20% (single) and 32% (couple) of an average adult full-time wage (1992–93).
- Over half of pensioner households depended on the state pension for at least 75% of their income (1991).
- The Department of Social Security suggests that a third of pensioners who are entitled to income support and a fifth entitled to housing benefit did not claim (1989).
- Older people of pensionable age spent more than twice the proportion of their outgoings on fuel, light and power as non-pensioner households (1991).

It is well established that pensioners spend more of their income on basic necessities such as fuel and food than others. Whereas full-time employee households spent 16% on food and 36% on fuel, retired households spent 21% of weekly household expenditure on food and 69% on fuel (Central Statistical Office 1995a). Many pensioners live in below standard housing. The vast majority (84%) of them have their homes colder than World Health Organization (WHO) recommendations. This has a direct relationship with the expense of heating (Age Concern 1995). Finally, pensioners living alone are more likely to suffer from a long term illness (Office of Population Censuses and Surveys 1993).

Unemployment

A further useful area to examine is the health of the unemployed. As an unemployed person, you are more likely to suffer from ill-health and also are more likely to die at an earlier age than those in paid employment (Morris et al 1994). Unemployment has consequently been recognised as a main cause of physical and mental ill-health (Moser et al 1984, Stern 1983).

Recent trends

Research suggests that inequalities in health are widening. Whitehead's (1987) update on inequalities in health in the 1980s pointed to a critical increase in health disparities throughout the decade. This has been validated in relation to increased disparity in mortality rates between the most deprived and the most affluent regional areas by Phillimore, Beattie and Townsend (Phillimore et al 1994).

Hence, as Blackburn (1994, p. 42) contends, low income 'acts as a key health hazard, increasing exposure to other health hazards … if the income "odds" are against you, then the likelihood is that other "odds" are also against you'.

ETHNIC GROUPS

So far we have discussed how health may be experienced by those of different economic status. Another form of stratification which affects our experience of health and illness is our ethnicity.

Ethnicity has been described as the most problematic form of social stratification (Reid 1989). This is due to the way ethnic groups are conceptualised and appear to operate in practice. As Reid (1989, p. 75) describes, 'While occupation is an easily understood and gathered piece of information for research purposes, ethnicity has a wide range of meanings and connotations'.

Many see ethnic groups as being defined by culturally distinctive ways of life. Barth (1969) has criticised the conventional wisdom that ethnic groups develop in isolation and has instead drawn attention to the importance of the boundaries that demarcate ethnic groups. He claims that it is the social interaction around these boundaries that helps to define these groups rather than their cultural content. Barth defined ethnic groups as categories of identification and ascription by the actors (people) themselves. People identify themselves and others as belonging to distinctive ethnic groups often on the basis of possessing certain key cultural criteria such as language, religion, customs and even dress. Cohen (1985), drawing on Barth's ideas, has defined ethnicity as 'the political assertion of cultural difference' distinguished by the individuals themselves.

Ethnic diversity in the UK

In spring 1995, there were 3.2 million people in Great Britain who classified themselves as belonging to a minority ethnic group, that is 6% of the total population (Office for National Statistics 1996). Just under half (45%) of this ethnic minority population lived in Greater London, with the conurbations of the West Midlands, West Yorkshire and the Greater Manchester areas also having significant ethnic minority populations. This contrasts with many rural areas where ethnic minorities form less than 1% of the population. Table 5.2 shows the composition of the ethnic minority population of Great Britain at the time of the 1991 census.

Apart from the ethnic groups outlined above, there are also a multitude of other smaller groups contributing to the cultural diversity of our modern society. It is crucial to appreciate the array of communities that are represented and not to imply commonality of experience within a general term of 'ethnic minorities' (Karmi 1993).

Equity Equity within a multicultural society has been described in the following way (definition by the National Association of Health Authorities, described in Karmi (1993)):

All people, irrespective of their religion, culture, race, colour, or ethnic background should have equal access to the NHS, should be offered services which are relevant and sensitive to their needs, should be able to use the NHS with confidence and expect to be

Table 5.2 The ethnic minority population of Great Britain, 1991 (after Ordnance Survey & HMSO 1995)

	Thousands	%
Black Caribbean	500	16.6
Black African	212	7.0
Black other	178	5.9
Indian	840	27.9
Pakistani	477	15.8
Bangladeshi	163	5.3
Chinese	157	5.2
Other Asian	198	6.6
Other non-Asian	290	9.6

treated with respect, should have equal rights of representation on NHS management bodies, and should have equality of opportunity in service provision and in NHS employment.

Health of ethnic minorities

Over recent years there has been an expanding literature on the health of ethnic minorities. One issue that is important to explore is the care that health care professionals provide for patients from ethnic minorities. Indeed, it has been argued (Karmi 1995) that health professionals' widespread unawareness concerning ethnic minority cultures and customs is one of the most unsatisfactory aspects of health care for ethnic minorities in Britain. Karmi argues that this ignorance has emanated from a dearth of instruction in multicultural health care during the training of health care professionals.

Health care professionals should aim to provide services which show an awareness of cultural variation. For example, the United Kingdom Central Council for Nursing, Midwifery and Health Visiting (UKCC), the regulatory body for registered nurses, midwives and health visitors, requires individual practitioners to 'take account of the customs, values and spiritual beliefs of patients' (UKCC 1993).

Issues in health care in a multicultural society

There are therefore a variety of issues that health care professionals need to be aware of. First of all, those providing health care need to be familiar with the dimensions and complexities involved in caring for people from diverse cultural backgrounds and meeting the needs of a multicultural society. The concepts of health and illness vary across different societies with traditional views on health and illness apparent in every ethnic group. Individual health beliefs are generally 'an amalgamation of cultural tradition, family tradition and personal education and experience' (Cook 1995, p. 24).

Issues of delivery and acceptance of health care need to be understood with consideration given to cultural difference, and to the issues

and barriers which one may come across in the working environment. Although various ethnic minority customs have no relation to health, several are acutely significant if ethnic groups are to receive culturally suitable and sensitive health care. For example some religious groups would find it unacceptable for female patients to be cared for by male health care professionals.

In addition, patterns of disease and illness vary between ethnic groups. A number of diseases, including heart disease, hypertension and diabetes, which affect all groups are none the less more prevalent in certain ethnic groups. Furthermore, inherited diseases specific to particular groups (for instance thalassaemia and sickle-cell anaemia) produce more differences (Karmi 1993). The impact of demographics on health care is consequently important and health care professionals need to understand this to enable more effective diagnosis and treatment.

Activities

- List some areas where health care professionals should be sensitive to the needs of people from ethnic minority groups.
- Carry out a literature search in your library on transcultural nursing and report to the rest of the class some of the more important findings.

INTERRELATIONSHIPS BETWEEN FACTORS

So far we have considered the impact on health of two forms of stratification, class which is partly the product of occupational status, and ethnicity. However, they do not have an effect independently, but instead they are often inextricably linked and can have a combined effect on an individual's experience of health and illness.

Ethnic groups and class

As an example, let us consider the link between ethnic groups and class. Statistics show that

Black and Asian people remain disadvantaged in terms of most social and economic indicators (Office for National Statistics 1996). Ethnic minorities generally fare considerably worse than the white population on the basis of pay, unemployment and housing. However, it is important to bear in mind that statistics do not paint a complete picture of ethnic minority lifestyles. They provide a general overview which can mask the diversity of experience.

Pay and employment   Consider the implications of the following statistics on income levels and occupational status (Office for National Statistics 1996):

- While the average hourly full-time rate is £6.59 for white women, it is as low as £4.78 for Pakistani/Bangladeshi women.
- The average hourly full-time rate for white men is £8.34 compared with £6.87 for Pakistani/Bangladeshi men.
- Unemployment is higher among all minority groups than among whites. For example, Black and Pakistani/Bangladeshi people have unemployment rates three times that of the white population.

Those from ethnic minorities are disproportionately represented in lower paid jobs, have less income, and therefore are in lower class or socioeconomic groups than white people. Many of the ethnic minority population, in particular those of Afro-Caribbean and Asian origin, are located within the ranks of the working class (Brown 1984). As a consequence they experience the class-shared determinants of poorer health and are more likely to experience the ill-health that accompanies the associated standards of living of poor housing, fewer amenities, and less access to appropriate health care.

Racial discrimination   It is also important to consider the impact of racial harassment and racism which can restrict employment opportunities, as well as access to housing and education. The structure of health services is also often unsuitable and promotes racial discrimination due to barriers to the uptake of and access to services through elements such as language barriers.

The nature of inequality

The nature of inequality should be examined by considering the combined impact of multiple factors which are tied up with every person's identity. For example, the experience of being an Asian professional woman living in Greater London compared to that of a white male skilled manual worker living in the East of Scotland may or may not be radically different.

Attempts to explain such different experiences can be complex. This complexity is a product of the interrelationships between the many social factors affecting our lives. As Reid (1989, p. 163) summarises: 'social and economic factors – including income, work and specific occupational health hazards, housing and environment, attitudes about health, lifestyle, and the provision, nature and use of health services – appear to be the basic ingredients within the interrelationship'.

ENVIRONMENT

The physical environment influences our experience of health, and impacts on well-being and quality of life. Examples of environmental determinants of health are air quality, concentrations of chemicals and substances in drinking water, noise levels, environmental protection and housing standards.

Environmental pollution

Using air quality as an example, it is possible to draw connections between levels of air pollution outdoors (due, for example, to traffic) and indoors (for example tobacco smoke) with levels of respiratory disease. Reductions in pollution and an increase in no smoking policies could greatly contribute to reduced respiratory distress and reducing health risks from environmental hazards.

UK national environmental health action plan

As part of the WHO initiative to improve environmental health, the Department of the

Environment launched its UK environmental health action plan in July 1996. This included 150 actions, including particular environmental hazards such as air and water pollution, and food contamination (Department of Health & Department of the Environment 1996). The UK plan will be used as a model for other European countries.

It is now likely that the government will announce that the environment will become the sixth key target of the Health of the Nation strategy (Department of Health 1992) with targets set for environmental factors such as air quality, noise pollution, and exposure to radon.

Distribution of health resources

A further environmental factor is the distribution of health resources. For example, Ordnance Survey & HMSO (1995) report that whereas the number of general practitioners (GPs) has been increasing and average patient size list has been falling, the distribution of GPs and size of patient lists across the UK does not correlate with the distribution of population. The report states that while the average number of people on a GP's list in Britain is 1870, in most regional health authority areas in England this figure is higher, in contrast to Scotland which had the smallest average size of lists. This pattern is broadly replicated for dentists.

There is also considerable regional variation in the provision of hospital care. An example is the proportion of people on waiting lists for over 1 year. Whereas Northern Ireland and Wales had the highest rates of 14% among those waiting for ordinary admissions, the lowest rate of 0.5% was in the Mersey Health Authority Area (Ordnance Survey & HMSO 1995).

Housing

Another significant environmental factor is the relationship between living conditions and health. The quality of housing has a significant impact on health. This association occurs because of factors such as defective design and inadequate maintenance, use of building materials such as asbestos, damp, insufficient lighting, sub-standard heating, and inferior sanitation.

A useful example concerns the rising number of cases of asthma that are seen to be the result of poor housing, in particular because of dampness. Since the 1980s, there has been a dramatic increase in the number of GP consultations and hospital admissions for asthma. In England alone asthma affects over 2 million people and is the cause of death for over 1600 people every year.

Local authority housing

The type of housing tenure can be a contributory factor to poor health. From information from the General Household Survey, Yuen, Machin and Balarajan (Yuen et al 1990) concluded that in comparison with tenants with other kinds of housing tenure, local authority tenants reported greater levels of ill-health. Blaxter (1990) describes evidence that suggests that the living environment in poorer areas is detrimental to health.

Towns and urban planning

Urban areas are often seen as prime examples of environmental degradation, with concentrations of poor housing, high unemployment and poverty. However, many rural areas may be characterised in similar ways. Indeed Harrison (1983 p. 21) has argued that the inner city is 'a microcosm of deprivation, of economic decline and of social disintegration' which are widespread across society.

Consequently it may be argued that environmental planning can be a contributor to health promotion (Krogh 1989). A clear method of outlining healthy town planning is to summarise the opposite (Krogh 1989, p. 97): 'Unhealthy town planning can help reduce people's chances to be physically and socially active. It can promote carelessness and alienation, leading to vandalism and violence. It can turn everyday functions into difficult and time-consuming activities, and it can add to pollution and other problems'. The converse of unhealthy or absent town planning would therefore serve to reverse these trends and promote improved well-being and quality of life.

LIFESTYLES AND BEHAVIOUR

It can be argued that we can make choices which affect our health, particularly in relation to our lifestyle and behaviour choices. However, choice should be viewed within its social context where conditions of low income and lack of resources act to restrict and impede choice. It may therefore be argued that lifestyle is economically determined, and that it would be misleading to detach individual conduct from the social context.

Smoking

A practical example of the impact of our habits on health is that of smoking. As *Social Trends* (Central Statistical Office, 1995b, p. 127) states: 'Smoking is the greatest cause of preventable death in this country and can lead to disease such as lung cancer, respiratory disease or heart disease. The Health Education Authority estimated that 110 thousand deaths in the United Kingdom in 1988 were attributable to smoking, representing about one in six deaths'.

Cigarette smoking has generally decreased among adults over the last few decades. For example, whereas in Great Britain, in 1972, 52% of men and 41% of women smoked cigarettes, in 1992, these figures had reduced to 29% of men and 28% of women (Central Statistical Office 1995b).

Smoking prevalence is recognised to vary between socioeconomic groups. It is worth noting that there are also gender differences. Whereas in 1992 14% of men and 13% of women in the professional group smoked cigarettes, this rises to 42% of men and 35% of women in the unskilled manual group. Therefore, men in the unskilled manual group are three times more likely to smoke than men in the professional group, with women displaying a similar though less striking pattern. Also, although there had been a decline in smoking prevalence in all socioeconomic groups, the most marked decline had been in non-manual groups rather than manual social groups. The net result is that these differences in smoking prevalence have extended over the last 20 years.

Smoking has been associated with severe disease such as cancer, particularly lung and oral cancer. The Ordnance Survey & HMSO (1995) asserted that 'smoking causes between 80 and 90% of lung cancer cases, with low levels of dietary antioxidants from fresh fruit and vegetables adding to this effect'. Death rates from oral cancer are three times higher in manual workers than in professional groups. The most significant risk factors are smoking and heavy alcohol consumption, particularly of spirits. The combined effect of alcohol and smoking appears to be greater than simply doubling the risk.

There are also regional differences in smoking prevalence, with the highest level of smoking in the UK for both men and women in Scotland. It should come as no surprise that areas with high levels of smoking, such as Scotland, have significant levels of smoking related cancers, and circulatory and respiratory diseases (Ordnance Survey & HMSO 1995).

Alcohol

'Alcohol consumption above sensible levels is thought to be associated with increased likelihood of social problems and ill health.' (Central Statistical Office 1995b, p. 129).

In 1992, nearly three in ten men (27%) and one in ten women (11%) drank more than the recommended maximum number of units per week (Central Statistical Office 1995b). Excessive alcohol consumption can contribute to ill-health such as liver disease, depression, some forms of cancer, and increase in accidents and injuries.

Patterns of expenditure

Income shapes health behaviour and therefore has an impact on quality of life. One useful guide to patterns of spending is the Family Expenditure Survey, a random survey of UK private households carried out by the Central Statistical

Office. After all, it is important not only to consider people's level of income but also the choices they make and the options available to them. The number of people in a household, their respective ages and other characteristics also affect spending.

The Family Expenditure Survey (Central Statistical Office 1995a) splits the population into ten income groups (decile groups). Table 5.3 shows the average weekly expenditure per person for all expenditure for each of these groups.

Concentrating on basic commodities such as food and fuel are helpful models, as health choices are linked to the amount of money to spend after fixed costs, such as housing and debts, are paid. From Table 5.4, it is clear that the lowest income 10% of the population spends a higher proportion of its income on commodities that might be defined as essential to subsistence.

Although expenditure on fuel and power rises with income, it represents a higher proportion of expenditure in lower income groups. Food ex-

penditure shows a similar pattern. For instance, the proportion of income spent on vegetables, potatoes and fresh fruit is broadly similar across all income groups, but in terms of actual money spent in different households, this represents £3.10 for the lowest income group compared with £10.60 within the highest income group. Therefore although different households are spending roughly equal proportions, because a household with a higher income may purchase a greater amount and variety of fresh fruit and vegetables the household will therefore be more likely to be able to secure good health.

Diet

Since the 1970s there have been significant alterations in the type of food eaten in the UK. We now eat more health, convenience and frozen foods. We eat more breakfast cereal, fewer eggs, less packet sugar and more fresh fruit, and there has been a considerable transfer from red meat to white meat.

However, the changes described above relate to average behaviour, and it is important to consider the variability between different social groups due to low income, choice and product availability.

Range of products available

First of all, consider the range of products available. During the period of intensive building programmes of the 1950s and 1960s in many major UK towns and cities, which created many large housing estates, little consideration was given to the provision of amenities such as shops. Therefore, for people living in these areas the choice of where to shop can be limited unless they are able to travel to supermarkets, shops and markets elsewhere.

Those on lower incomes are least likely to live in areas that have reasonably priced outlets for fresh foods (Glasgow Healthy City Project 1992). With superstores often difficult to travel to without access to a private car, many are unable to take advantage of cheaper goods. Lack of transport can also prohibit being able to

Table 5.3 Average weekly expenditure per person for all expenditure (£) by gross income decile group (after Central Statistical Office 1995a)

Decile group	(£)
Lowest decile group	67.50
Second decile group	62.66
Third decile group	72.76
Fourth decile group	88.35
Fifth decile group	105.77
Sixth decile group	109.45
Seventh decile group	119.38
Eighth decile group	125.74
Ninth decile group	140.69
Tenth decile group	195.40
All households	116.95

Table 5.4 Household expenditure as a percentage of total expenditure by gross income decile group (after Central Statistical Office 1995a)

	Housing (net)	Fuel and power	Food and non-alcoholic drink
Lowest 10%	14.7	10.9	25.5
Highest 10%	16.4	3.0	14.3

purchase large quantities at cheaper prices. Storage space within the home is also significant as being without adequate cupboard space and, for example, a freezer, makes it impossible to take advantage of bulk purchasing and means that more shopping trips may need to be made.

Choice

Also consider the element of choice within households. In many households the choice of food and method of preparation by one individual affects the patterns of food consumption for the rest of the household.

Cost

It has been claimed that a healthy diet costs more than an inadequate one (Leather 1992). The additional expense required for a healthy diet appears to penalise those on low incomes, such as those on state benefits. Rather than supporting the view that those on low incomes are buying unwisely, Leather argues that for most people a healthy diet is unrealisable without going into debt or reducing money spent on other basic essentials.

Low cost local initiatives However, there are many local initiatives around the UK aimed at resolving this situation. In some areas initiatives such as not-for-profit food shops for those on low incomes have been undertaken to create a wider range of fresh produce at reasonable prices to local residents. An example is that within the Bingham area of Edinburgh, an area of deprivation and poor housing which was demolished in the late 1980s and new housing built. Here a local cooperative was set up by residents to buy fresh produce and sell to Bingham residents at low prices to improve the range of products available and improve the health of the area.

Health consequences

The health consequences of an inadequate diet range from poor nutrition and lower heights to shortened life expectancy of those from lower income families. A limited diet with inferior

nutritional value commonly follows a restricted budget.

It has been argued that adopting a healthy lifestyle within a favourable social environment matters, whereas a healthy lifestyle within an unfavourable social environment does not make much difference in health (Blaxter 1990). Blaxter (1990) seeks to argue that social and material circumstances therefore outweigh the benefits to be gained from a healthy lifestyle.

Activities

- Describe how the government has discouraged smoking.
- Discuss with your friends how the government targets specific societal groups in anti-smoking campaigns.
- Make a list of ideas that would support the government's current anti-smoking policies.

INEQUALITIES IN HEALTH

'Inequalities in health are of concern to the whole nation and represent one of the biggest possible challenges to the conduct of government policy.' (Townsend et al 1992, p. 1).

The underlying explanations for varying health chances appear to point towards a variety of social factors. As Moore & Harrisson (1995, p. 222) suggest, many of these may be viewed as 'proxy indicators for economic status'. The varying experience between individuals and groups of health and illness can be described as inequalities in health.

Following concentrated academic and political debate on health inequalities, a research working group on inequalities in health, chaired by Sir Douglas Black, was formed by the government to investigate the issues. The group's report became known as the Black Report (DHSS 1980).

The report validated prevailing class differences in health, confirming that those in lower social classes experienced persistent poorer health. It also acknowledged that the predicament went beyond health services and transcended many socioeconomic factors, all of which were connected by income. These included unemployment, housing, environment, transport and education.

The remedy to these problems put forward by the Black Report was far reaching social reform. To improve the health of the nation, the focus would have to be on tackling social deprivation and poverty. The Black Report proved a catalyst for debate and future research on disparities in health which has focused on linking health chances to social factors and the association between wealth and health.

Activities

- List some reasons why the government was hesitant when releasing the findings of the Black Report (DHSS 1980).
- Form a group and discuss the value of the Black Report in the context of social policy.

EQUITY

A central issue is equity of service provision and utilisation of health care services. Titmuss (1968) outlined significant disparities between those of different income levels. Those with lower incomes received fewer health services and accessed less than those who had higher incomes who were able to make greater use of available services. For example, those in higher income groups received greater levels of specialist care, and were more likely to attend GPs than those of lower incomes.

It has also been suggested that people with different incomes receive different responses and treatment from medical professionals (Blaxter 1984). The situation of those who are in most need receiving the lowest proportion of health care has been described as the inverse care law (Hart 1971).

Explanations for unequal provisions and access are complex and related to knowledge, availability of resources such as use of a private telephone or car, and available time to spend on health.

Draper (1989) describes two dimensions to the equity debate. Firstly, ethical queries about what makes up equal opportunity and fairness, plus the practicality of harmonising equity with competing demands which are often economic. Indeed economic arguments are commonly used to explain why equity is not pursued.

If health needs differ, it can be argued that health services should target those in greater need and be made easier to access for the disadvantaged in society. As Whitehead (1991 p. 220) contends 'equity is therefore concerned with creating equal opportunities for health and with bringing health differentials down to the lowest level possible'. To do so requires multi-agency co-operation.

SOCIAL MODEL OF HEALTH PRACTICE

Preventable health disparities

Certain determinants of health disparities can be viewed as preventable. Whitehead (1991, p. 219) describes such elements as 'health damaging behaviour where the degree of choice of lifestyles is severely restricted' and 'exposure to unhealthy, stressful living and working conditions'. Whitehead describes other elements where the focus is on low income which seems preventable and unfair. These include 'inadequate access to essential health and other public services' and 'natural selection or health-related social mobility involving the tendency for sick people to move down the social scale'.

Initiatives

Initiatives can be devised to address the imbalanced relationship between different social groups and health care. This can include plans to avoid restricted choice and exposure to unhealthy environments, and also to tackle difficulties stemming from low incomes. Initiatives can range from government policy to local projects which health care professionals can facilitate in their area of work.

Economic approaches

Models favoured by the political left to address 'the cumulative effect of the different elements of material deprivation' (Morris & Harrisson 1995), and consequently improve health in a society, focus on ensuring the most equal distribution of wealth through redistribution. From this viewpoint only through improving the economic state of those with low incomes can progress be made towards improving their health.

An alternative view, such as that behind many of the measures within the UK during the 1980s and 1990s, is that the best way to improve health is to increase the overall wealth of the society. However, there is evidence to suggest that this latter approach has led to increased inequalities within society, including health inequalities.

Multi-agency approach

Breaking the cycle between poverty and ill-health requires a multi-agency approach, including long term commitment from housing, health and public works to community-based health initiatives and development.

Healthy Cities Project The WHO Healthy Cities Project is an example of social policy designed to address the disparities in health status between different social groups. The principle that all people have an equal right to health is the foundation of the project. The activities promoted by this initiative focus on altering the social and physical environment, providing the means to support healthy lifestyles, and ensuring services are available to all.

Changing the physical and social environment requires broad policies aimed at structural

Activities

- Find out what the city council nearest to where you live is doing in support of the Healthy Cities Project.
- Investigate some of the projects that have been undertaken in major cities like Edinburgh, Glasgow, Dublin and Belfast in support of the Healthy Cities Project.

developments in working and living environments. Policies to enable healthy lifestyles centre on reducing lifestyle risks through health education combined with treating the fundamental conditions affecting lifestyle. Action to ensure that services are accessible to all should concentrate on eliminating barriers to services, whether they be cultural, organisational, financial or environmental.

Health for All Another WHO strategy is that of *Health for All* (WHO 1985), which is based on the principle of equity. As Touros (1989, p. 73) describes, 'This target [of equity] could be achieved if the basic prerequisites for health (such as food, shelter, secure work and a useful role in society) were provided for all, if the risks related to lifestyle were reduced, if the health aspects of living and working conditions were improved (by creating physical and social environments conducive to health) and if good continuous care were accessible to all'. The targets promoted by the WHO present challenges for politicians and those in positions of power to achieve reductions in social differences in health while promoting equal health opportunities for all (Touros 1989).

The Health of the Nation *The Health of the Nation: a strategy for health*, was launched by the UK government in 1992 to address key elements affecting the country's health (Department of Health 1992). Specific targets were set to improve health in five key areas such as cancer and mental illness. The aims are 'adding years to life by reducing premature death and increasing life expectancy; while adding life to years: increasing years lived free from ill-health, reducing or minimising the adverse effects of illness and disability, promoting healthy lifestyles, physical and social environments and, overall, improving quality of life' (Department of Health 1992).

The ideology behind this policy rejects the view that health and lifestyle may be economically determined, and has instead stressed the importance of individuals changing their behaviour. By concentrating on individual behaviour the strategy has failed so far to address many of the structural issues such as low income and poverty which directly affect health. The strategy has therefore been criticised for failing to adequately address inequalities in health (Davey-Smith & Morris 1994).

However, despite these criticisms, the strategy shapes many areas of current practice for health care professionals. Indeed the government established that 'Success in key areas [of the Health of the Nation] will depend greatly on the commitment and skills of family and community doctors, nurses, midwives and health visitors' (Department of Health 1992). An example is the area of dietary change where an appropriate social model would focus on understanding the barriers to healthy eating. Practical methods could then be pursued with an emphasis on improving rather than constructing an ideal diet.

The effect of social policies

Draper (1989) provides examples of social policies which can maintain or increase inequalities and contrasts these with examples of policies which can lessen inequalities.

Policies that reinforce inequalities in health status include (Draper 1989, p. 92):

- municipal building programmes that do not provide access for older or disabled people
- the failure to control air, water and noise pollution in low-income neighbourhoods
- housing codes that do not take the needs of the elderly into account
- limited access to day care for single-parent families
- policies on basic education that limit access for groups such as women, functionally illiterate adults or minority groups
- the denial of access to birth control and abortion services
- the failure to provide employment opportunities suited to the abilities of the disabled
- health education programmes that deal with lifestyle without addressing environmental factors
- the provision of health services only in the language of major population groups
- the denial of sickness benefits and other social security benefits to migrant workers.

These suggestions not only concentrate on the provision of health services but also on factors which impact on health chances such as employment, education, environment and access to benefits. Compare the above list with the examples of policies that Draper (1989, pp. 92–3) offers to reduce inequalities (below).

Policies that reduce inequalities in health status include:

- the provision of social security benefits for older people and the disabled offering an income sufficient to provide essentials for living
- the encouragement of community and neighbourhood participation in decisions about housing and urban planning
- the adoption of health education programmes that address environmental as well as lifestyle issues
- the provision of universal free education, with special emphasis on access for disadvantaged groups and linguistic and ethnic minorities
- housing designs that are easily fitted to meet the needs of frail older people and the disabled
- equal opportunity employment policies for the disabled and for minority groups
- labour policies that encourage flexibility, variety and self-determination in the workplace
- the provision of easy access to day-care services with priority for single-parent families
- the introduction of programmes to protect the relative position of the disadvantaged during periods of economic decline
- the provision of primary health care services in the languages of minority groups, with easy access for people with limited education
- vigorous enforcement of human rights codes.

You will notice that many of the suggested policies in the second list are opposites of those in the previous list, and that they also cover a wide range of social factors. Therefore action which may be taken to reduce the effects of social issues on health are not only limited to health initiatives, but can be expanded to policies affecting the wide range of social factors which influence our health.

Many of the suggested policies could be viewed as controversial, considering the challenge they present to existing structures. Draper (1989) argues that to generate the political will and public support necessary to enable these policies to succeed, 'policy relevant knowledge, an effective forum for policy advocacy, an infrastructure for policy formation and processes to encourage planning and action' are all required.

Local strategies

So far discussion has centred on large scale initiatives and policies to improve health. Social models of health practice may also be designed by health care professionals at the local level to address particular issues within an area. The following examples of health profiling and promoting equality for ethnic groups provide suggestions of how registered nurses can adopt strategies aimed at tackling the effect of social issues and health. Registered nurses have been chosen as a sample group as around 80% of direct patient care is provided by nurses, midwives and health visitors, with nursing services forming close to a quarter of the NHS budget.

Health profiling   Health profiling can be seen as the first step towards incorporating a social model into nursing practice. A health profile compiled for a specific population can be placed within the care environment, such as the general practice, a school, or an accident and emergency department, or it can be focused on a cultural or geographical population. The Royal College of Nursing (RCN) (1996a) outlines four basic principles of health profiling:

- collecting and analysing information
- selecting priorities for action
- choosing nursing activities, including methods of working, for selected priorities
- evaluating nursing practice.

Information will vary according to local circumstance but should be gathered on 'incidence of disease, illness, disability and trauma; information on health service provision, for example,

immunisation uptake; social and environmental data such as housing, occupation, receipt of welfare benefits' (RCN 1994). The views of patients or clients and those of health care professionals and other key workers are also important. Specific guidance has been published on health profiling, providing a detailed framework for members of the primary health care team (RCN 1993).

Once information has been gathered it can be analysed to identify and select priorities. Priorities can be aimed at individuals, at a group or community level, or at a national and/or local campaign level. Appropriate nursing activities can then be chosen to pursue appropriate action. As many initiatives are dependent on a multi-agency approach, it will be important to coordinate activity with others such as social workers, environmental health officers or voluntary workers. An evaluation of nursing practice will assist in the development of future action. The following presents a summary of suggestions for key activities:

- assess the health needs of local populations through compilation of health profiles
- support people to participate in the life of their community to influence factors which affect their health
- build healthy alliances and a supportive infrastructure to provide information, resources and practical help for community initiatives
- increase health resources in communities by establishing local networks
- engage with the local statutory and voluntary groups to work towards health related policies and actions
- increase uptake of health services by ensuring they are accessible, offered appropriately and effectively targeted.

Poverty profiling   An essential part of health profiling should be the identification of measures of poverty (RCN 1996a). The basic principles of profiling outlined above can be applied. Profiling poverty within a community or particular care population can enable registered nurses to clarify the relationships between poverty and health status in their local area. This knowledge can then provide the means by which registered nurses can plan, target, deliver and audit nursing services to ensure appropriate provision. It can also provide supporting evidence for requests for additional health resources and resources from other statutory agencies.

Health strategies for ethnic groups Health practice directed at particular divisions in society provides further examples of local social models. A practical strategy that registered nurses can pursue are policies which aim to improve the experiences of ethnic groups. The following steps, taken from a guide for nurses on contracting for race and health equality (RCN 1996b), could be pursued to promote equality of opportunity and the avoidance of racial discrimination.

- Hold regular consultation meetings on the [equal opportunity] policy with nursing staff and other health workers as well as representatives of service users.
- Offer training and guidance for nursing staff and other health workers on the implications of the policy for service provision and for individual action programmes.
- Cooperate with nursing staff and other health workers on devising race equality objectives for the following year. For example nursing staff may identify that maternity service users would benefit from an improved advocacy service.
- Plan and implement a training programme to ensure that relevant staff understand the need for ethnic record keeping.
- Appropriate dietary advice and provision which takes account of cultural and religious background.
- Health education which is relevant to users' cultural and religious background.
- Clinical audit which monitors the particular vulnerability of minority ethnic communities to specific illness patterns.

Summary

Social characteristics exert a powerful sway on our quality of life and our likelihood of experiencing ill-health or contracting severe disease. Evidence suggests that health chances are socially determined through the interrelationship of factors with the cumulative effect having critical ramifications for health.

While in absolute terms it may be argued that standards of living and lifestyles have improved throughout the latter part of the 20th century with effects on individual health chances, the relative differences inherent in our society have remained between those who have access to economic security and those who do not. Indeed some commentators have argued that relative differences between social groups have in fact grown. From the considerable evidence confirming that health can be socially determined, it is clear that structural problems such as poverty and income inequality have to be addressed.

This chapter has identified some of the social factors which can affect people's experience of health and illness, and has explored the complex relationships between social issues and health. The issues identified include class and occupational status, ethnic groups, poverty, environment, lifestyles and behaviour. Consideration has been given to the effect these factors have on health chances, inequalities in health and equity. Finally, social models of health practice have been described and suggestions made of action which health care professionals can undertake to challenge the effect of social issues on health.

Activities

- Select a current health promotion issue and list ten strategies that the government has utilised to encourage positive behaviour.
- Organise a debate with your friends and discuss whether it is appropriate that economic resources should focus on either treating ill-health or health promoting and preventive strategies.
- Carry out a literature search in your library to find evidence of the benefits of health promotion campaigns.

REFERENCES

Age Concern England 1995 Short change. Age Concern, London

Barth F 1969 Ethnic groups and boundaries. Little Brown, Boston

Blackburn C 1994 Low income, inequality and health promotion. Nursing Times 90(90):42–43

Blaxter M 1984 Equity and consultation rates in general practice. British Medical Journal 288:1963–1967

Blaxter M 1990 Health and lifestyle. Tavistock/Routledge, London

Brown C 1984 Black and white. Policy Studies Institute/ Heinemann Educational, Oxford

Central Statistical Office 1995a Family expenditure: a report on the 1994–5 family expenditure survey. HMSO, London

Central Statistical Office 1995b Social trends 25. HMSO, London

Cohen T 1985 The symbolic construction of community. Routledge, London

Cook R 1995 Immunisation: creating the culture. Practice Nursing 6(8):23–24

Davey-Smith G, Morris J 1994 Increasing inequalities in the health of the nation. British Medical Journal 309:1453–1454

Department of Health and Social Security 1980 Inequalities in health: report of a research working group chaired by Sir Douglas Black. DHSS, London

Department of Health 1992 The Health of the Nation: a strategy for health for England. HMSO, London

Department of Health, Department of the Environment 1996 United Kingdom national environmental health action plan. HMSO, London

Draper R 1989 Making equity policy. Health Promotion 4(2):91–95

Giddens A 1993 Sociology, 2nd edn. Polity Press, Cambridge

Glasgow Healthy City Project 1992 Conference paper. Cited in: George M 1993 Nursing Standard 7(49):21–32

Harrison P 1983 Inside the inner city: life under the cutting edge. Penguin, Harmondsworth

Hart J T 1971 The inverse care law. Lancet 271(7696): 405–412

Karmi G 1993 Equity and health of ethnic minorities. Quality in Health Care 2(2):100–103

Karmi G 1995 The ethnic health handbook: a factfile for health care professionals. Blackwell Science, London

Krogh L 1989 Trends in town planning in the 1980s: equity and healthy planning. Health Promotion 4(2):97–101

Leather S 1992 Your food: whose choice. National Consumer Council, London

Mitchell J 1984 What is to be done about illness and health? Penguin, London

Montgomery L E, Carter-Pokras O 1993 Health status by social class and/or minority status: implications for environmental equity research. Toxicology and Industrial Health 9(5):729–773

Moore R, Harrisson S 1995 In poor health: socioeconomic status and health chances – a review of the literature. Social Sciences and Health 1(4):221–235

Morris J K, Cook D G, Shaper A G 1994 Loss of employment and mortality. British Medical Journal 308:1135–1139

Moser K A, Fox A J, Jones D R 1984 Unemployment and mortality in the OPCS longitudinal study. Lancet 2(8415): 1324–1329

Najman J M 1993 Health and poverty: past, present and prospects for the future. Social Science Medical Journal 36(2):157–166

Office for National Statistics 1989 Standard occupational classification (soc.) volume 1, HMSO, London

Office for National Statistics 1996 Social focus on ethnic minorities. HMSO, London

Office of Population Censuses and Surveys 1993 Limiting long-term illness. OPCS, London

Ordnance Survey, HMSO 1995 Statlas UK: a statistical analysis of the United Kingdom. HMSO, Southampton

Phillimore P, Beattie A, Townsend P 1994 Widening inequality of health in Northern England, 1981–1991. British Medical Journal 308:1125–1128

Reid I 1989 Social class difference in Britain: life chances and lifestyles, 3rd edn. Fontana, Glasgow

Royal College of Nursing 1993 The GP practice population profile. RCN, London

Royal College of Nursing 1994 Public health: nursing rises to the challenge. RCN, London

Royal College of Nursing 1996a Profiling poverty: a guide for nurses in the community. RCN, London

Royal College of Nursing 1996b Contracting for race and health equality: a guide for the nursing profession. RCN, London

Stern J 1983 The relationship between unemployment, morbidity and mortality in Britain. Population Studies 37:61

Teale C 1996 Money problems and financial help. British Medical Journal 313(3):288–290

Titmuss R M 1968 Commitment to welfare. Allen and Unwin, London

Touros A D 1989 Equity and the Healthy Cities project. Health Promotion 4(2):73–75

Townsend P 1979 Poverty in the United Kingdom. Penguin, London

Townsend P, Davidson N, Whitehead M 1992 Inequalities in health: the Black Report and the health divide. Penguin, London

United Kingdom Central Council for Nursing, Midwifery and Health Visiting 1993 Code of Conduct. UKCC, London

Webster C 1991 Aneurin Bevan on the National Health Service. University of Oxford Wellcome Unit for the History of Medicine, Oxford

Whitehead M 1987 The health divide: inequalities in health in the 1980s. Education Council, London

Whitehead M 1991 The concepts and principles of equity and health. Health Promotion International 6(3):217–228

World Health Organization 1985 Targets for health for all. WHO Regional Office for Europe, Copenhagen

Yuen P, Machin D, Balarajan R 1990 Inequalities in health: socioeconomic differences in self-reported morbidity. Public Health 104:65–71

Gender issues

Siân P. Thomas

At the end of this chapter the reader should be able to:

- **outline some theories of gender**
- **explore gender issues in relation to health care**
- **explore the relationship between gender and health chance**
- **outline the social construction of caring and health work as a gendered occupation within the wider sphere of gender and work**

Introduction

This chapter explores key issues that surround the area of gender and its association with health care provision. It aims to introduce readers to some of the theories that attempt to explain why there are divisions in society that are based on gender. From this premise the chapter will go on to examine the relationship between gender and health chances and the different health experiences of men and women. In working through this chapter it is hoped that the readers' own beliefs and practices will emerge in terms of how they feel about gender as an issue and its relation to health care.

GENDER DIFFERENCES

An understanding of how men and women are socially constructed provides a starting point for any discussion regarding the cultural issue of gender, rather than focusing on inherent physiological differences. A simple difference between women and men as social categories exists in most countries and societies. For the most part it is used as a means of linking the cultural values that are given to the categories of 'woman' and 'man', and to the organisation of men's and women's activities in society. For example, the concept of 'mother' is a cultural construct which different cultures elaborate in different ways (Moore 1988). In Western society, the categories 'woman' and 'mother' overlap, leading to a definition of woman which is dependent on the idea of a 'mother' and the association of activities that this maternal concept draws, such as caring and tending. This 'natural' association can, however, be questioned because there is variability across cultures, both in the composition of domestic groups and in the arrangements whereby particular individuals are assigned to the task of child rearing. Within British society this can be illustrated by reference to changing ideas about motherhood, childhood and family life over the last century, with gender divisions and perceptions of suitable gender roles varying over time and because of political events such as economic crises or conflicts and wars.

Bio-psychological

A biological approach to the gender argument usually begins with biological reproduction and motherhood. Women are considered to be more home centred and because it is women who give birth to children, it is thought by many that they should have a greater responsibility in meeting children's needs. A second biological factor is connected to differences in physical make-up other than biological function. This argument is based on different genetic features; for example women are generally smaller and so men are generally considered to be stronger. This view is, however, fraught with inconsistencies because of the variations that obviously exist in physical attributes among men and women. It also ignores social and cultural factors that are vital to any appreciation of gender. From a psychological perspective, gender centres on the development of the human psyche and is associated with the ideas of Freud and subsequent psychoanalysts. This theory, based on descriptive values, is important for understanding how gender divisions operate, particularly regarding the origins of power relations. However, because the differences are not peculiar to either gender the reliability of a single dimension argument can be questioned.

Sociological

A distinction has been made between sex and gender, particularly in early feminist literature. Sex is based on biological differences associated with reproduction, while gender is centred on socially created distinctions and is dependent on cultural differences. The topic of gender is commonly debated as a social construct that is linked to upbringing and other concepts such as self, personhood and autonomy. From this perspective, the connections that exist between symbolic or cultural aspects of social life and the economic and social conditions in which life is lived are made clear. Enquiry and analysis of gender identity is an area where feminist theorists continue to make a significant contribution to the theoretical development of the social science disciplines. Particularly among 'symbolic interactionist' theorists, gender issues are examined as a symbolic issue because it is in the context of particular social and economic relationships that cultural ideas of gender have emerged (Collier and Rosaldo in Ortner & Whitehead 1981). In contrast, sociologists who take a functionalist view argue that gender divisions are social in origin and that the separation of the roles of men and women is functionally necessary for society. A key functionalist theorist, Parsons (1955), proposed that the nuclear family unit is ideal to meet the needs of a mature industrial capitalist economy. With the husband as breadwinner and the wife as homemaker, the nuclear family unit nurtures men in preparation for paid work outside the home and performs the socialisation of children in readiness for the next generation to continue this cycle.

Marxist perspectives contain a functionalist element by tracing the subordination of women to the economic system and therefore attempting to account for gender differences through the capitalist economic system. Women's oppression is linked to economic production, which is exploitative in class terms. Engels's view was that the subordination of women has its roots in the institution of private property. Private property persists through inheritance, for which paternity is significant. The control of women's sexuality therefore becomes paramount in order that paternity can be traced and inheritance maintained. However, this is only of relevance to those who hold private property (the bourgeois class). The subordination of women in other classes is simply written off as a relic of pre-capitalist systems. For those who espouse a Marxist view, the emancipation of women can be realised in terms of equality, by joining in the class struggle.

Activities

- Discuss with your colleagues the effects of biological difference as a factor in gender divisions In society.
- Organise a debate with your colleagues to discuss the role of women in Britain from a functionalist perspective.

THE FEMINIST APPROACH

Liberal feminists

A feminist approach has been described as a means of examining 'differences between the power, social position, attitudes and behaviour of men and women ... putting forward theories to account for them and exploring ways in which current practices in society might be changed ... to release women from their subordination' (Women and Geography Study Group 1984, p. 25). Liberal feminist theory of gender division accepts some functionalist elements but introduces the notion of inequality. Those sharing this viewpoint are committed to promoting greater equality by the fairer division of tasks and the re-evaluation of tasks. Equal

opportunities for men and women are stressed. The activities generally associated with women (for example the care of children) are stressed as important tasks in contemporary society and it is considered that they should be more highly valued. The liberal feminist strategy is therefore one of equality and re-evaluation of what women do, with an emphasis on placing equal value on these tasks rather than supporting difference between women and men.

Radical feminists

In contrast to the liberal view, radical feminists perceive gender as a fundamental division in society from which other differences are created, including race and class. When these are combined with gender it produces a complex pattern of dominance and subordination. The subordination of women by men is therefore seen as the fundamental inequality in all human societies. The idea of patriarchy is central to radical feminism. This refers to any system of male domination as a set of social relations between men, which allows them to dominate women. The basis of patriarchal power is men's ability to control what kinds of work women do through control of economic and social institutions and through the perpetuation of beliefs and attitudes which account for men's dominance in society. It is from this premise that Millet (1971) takes the view that every avenue of power is entirely in male hands and women's work is confined to the 'private' sphere of carrying out child rearing and personal and sexual services for men.

Radical feminists also see women's control over their own sexuality and bodies as being controlled by men. Medical services provide a useful example, in terms of accessing and availability of contraception, abortion, pre- and postnatal care. In Firestone's view (1971), the key factor in women's oppression lies in women's inherent restriction caused by the reproductive function of pregnancy. Other radical feminists emphasise rape and sexual violence as mechanisms of gender relations (Brownmillar 1975), while others take the view that the marriage contract is the key origin of gender division (Delphy 1984).

Socialist feminists

Socialist feminists provide yet another interpretation. They link gender relations to the wider framework of social relations which are structured by other factors as well as gender differences. They reject the notion that gender divisions are the fundamental division and instead see the mechanism of labour and class as the primary source of division. Socialist feminists also take a flexible view towards the distribution of gender divisions. First they contend that oppression is not unique to capitalism and second, they suggest that the level or degree of division varies between different sections of society. Socialist feminists take a more conciliatory line towards the position of men in society. Rather than seeing men as the enemy, like radical feminists for example, socialist feminists propose that men and women should unite in class struggle.

Gender relations and typing

The term gender relations is used to describe the different dynamics that operate between men and women. It is quite common for roles to be reversed at an individual level, to reflect individual views as to appropriate behaviour or activities between a man and women. However, within the broad patterns of gender relations typified in UK society there is little evidence of significant changes in roles. An example of gender roles and sex typing is the social allocation of tasks to women and men, for example caring and nurturing roles to women, and leadership roles to men. Sex typing therefore refers to a task typed by sex. For example, the word 'nurse' takes on a female connotation for many people in the same way that 'engineer' takes on a male connotation. This division is one of the most important ways of organising society and one which is strengthened by the unequal distribution of power and influence.

The vast majority of women are economically dependent on men. The reasons for this relate to low wages, recruitment and work practices and domestic demands that limit women's employment prospects. Women also fulfil a dual role of paid work and domestic work. Male domination operates at two levels. At a macro level it limits women's immediate and long term opportunities through male control of organisations, situations and their rules. At the micro level, domination is continued through family, work and social relations. Zaretsky (1976) recognises the separation between waged work and domestic work and contends that men are oppressed by waged work and women are oppressed by being excluded from waged work and secluded in the home within the private environment.

It has been argued by Dalla Costa & James (1975) that housework is essential for capitalism to reproduce the labour force and, as a hidden and unpaid form of waged work, it is therefore maximising capitalist profit. In Dalla Costa & James's view, women should demand wages for housework rather than working (paid) and doing housework for free which imposes a double working day. In this debate Marxist approaches have also been criticised for ignoring gender inequality in non-capitalist economies, particularly in terms of the benefits men gain from women's further oppression.

Activities

- Discuss the various strands of the feminist debate and outline the key differences and similarities.
- Consider your own views and position in the debate, make brief notes on your views and discuss them with colleagues.

INEQUALITY IN HEALTH CARE

Inequalities between men and women are reflected in the organisation of health care in the UK. Views about appropriate behaviour, occupations and so on for women and men seem to influence the treatment individuals receive in health care and lead to inequality in provision. Unfortunately these negative and biased attitudes are often presented as 'common sense' or 'part of our culture'. Each culture has attitudes about gender and because it is part of a culture these attitudes can be difficult to dispute. This can be a difficult issue for those providing health care because they will also have additional views about men and women. When cultural and personal attitudes are combined this can lead to differential treatment based on negative views. Further inequalities such as class, race, disability, age and sexual orientation only compound these negative perspectives towards women. Williams (1989) presents the view that most components of the welfare state are part of a racially structured and patriarchal capitalism system. Williams goes on to contend that gender and race are marginalised in the discipline of social policy, and proposes that substantial movement needs to take place towards a more integrated and inclusive approach. Being alert to how power inequalities exist within the differing attitudes of health care professionals and within health service provision enables unfair and inappropriate care to be challenged.

Activity

Read through some chapters from Fiona Williams's critique of the welfare state (Williams 1989), then consider with your colleagues whether inequalities could exist in an area of public service, such as housing, health or personal and social services.

GENDER AND HEALTH CHANCES

It is possible to examine the divisions in society between men and women by exploring differences in health experiences. Over the last century there have been substantial gains in life expectancy. Projected mortality rates for 1996 show that a boy born in that year can expect to live until he is 74 while a girl can expect to live until she is nearly 80 (Central Statistics Office 1995). There is, however, a common misconception that this is the result of an extension in the expected life span, whereas the real reason lies in the fact that a larger number of individuals now survive childhood. The infectious diseases which predominated in childhood among previous gener-

ations have been eliminated. The leading causes of death today are chronic diseases, especially heart disease and cancers, both of which have been shown to have a growing gender bias.

The relationship between gender and health is not straightforward. Inherent are the different dimensions of inequality which combine to produce health chances for each individual's set of circumstances. For example research studies have shown a link between smoking, motherhood and material circumstances. Graham (1995) describes a study of smoking behaviour amongst working class women which links cigarette smoking to additional caring responsibilities and restricted access to material resources (including recreational and social support networks). A further example is material inequality in later life contributing to ill-health. From a gender perspective, the ageing population of the UK has an increasing gender imbalance of more older women than older men. In addition there is a growing proportion of older women living alone. Material inequality in later life can be analysed in relation to differences in income from roles during earlier life stages. As many older women have been economically dependent on men throughout their life cycle, many are less likely to have pension security and sufficient material resources.

The General Household Survey

The General Household Survey (GHS) is a continuous survey based on a sample of the general population resident in private households in Great Britain. It is carried out by the Social Survey Division within the Office of Population Censuses and Surveys (OPCS). The GHS provides a means of examining relationships between a wide range of variables with which social policy is concerned, including questions on population and fertility, housing, health, employment and education. In particular, it paints a broad picture of people's lives and monitors a number of trends and changes over time. For example the 1994 survey included information on the characteristics of the population, reported smoking and drinking behaviour, health and GP consultations, and older people (OPCS 1996).

Respondents were asked about their current health and long-standing illness, for which the most common causes were disorders of the musculoskeletal system, problems of the heart and circulatory system, and respiratory problems. Different experiences were reported by class, age and gender. For example there was a higher reported prevalence of musculoskeletal problems among women, while men aged between 45 and 74 were more likely to report circulatory or heart problems than women in the same age group. Women were more likely to report suffering from hypertension and arthritis, while men were more likely to report a heart attack than women.

Patterns of health service use

As well as differences in health problems, there are apparent patterns in the use of health services by men and women. First of all let us look at the example of GP consultations. (This relates to GP consultations only and not the wider provision of primary care services such as other services provide by general practices, for example the increasing use of practice nurses to run specialised clinics.) The self-reported health of the general population based on individuals' perceptions of their own health and illness is more meaningful than more objective measures of prevalence when it comes to demand for health services

Throughout the 1980s there was an increase, particularly among women, of those reporting to have consulted their GP. 'In 1981, 10% of males and 14% of females, reported a GP consultation compared with 13% and 18% respectively in 1995' (Office for National Statistics Social Survey Division 1997). Women are more likely to consult their GPs than men, with the largest differences in consultation use being within the 16–44 age group, where 18% of women consulted their GP compared with 10% of men. Many visits related to reproductive health, such as pregnancy, and contraceptive advice may also contribute to this pattern.

Activities

- List six reasons why women tend to smoke more than in previous decades
- List six reasons why women are more likely to visit their GPs than men
- Organise a seminar to share some of these findings with your colleagues

HEALTH PROMOTION AND EDUCATION

Within the NHS there has been a changing emphasis from a curing service to one that promotes health and actively seeks to prevent illness. Health promotion and patient education have been shown to play a valuable role in influencing health-related knowledge, attitudes and behaviour in both men and women. The *Health of the Nation* White Paper in 1992 identified five key areas where there was the greatest need and scope for improvements in health of people in England. Similar targets were prepared for Scotland and Wales. Key areas were coronary heart disease and stroke, cancers, mental illness, HIV/AIDS and sexual health, and accidents. Risk factors were identified from these key areas, including smoking, alcohol, diet and nutrition, obesity, blood pressures and HIV/AIDS.

The Health Education Authority in England developed health promotion indicators to measure intermediate progress in these key results areas. The Social Survey Division of the Office of National Statistics has carried out two health education monitoring surveys for the Health Education Authority in England to monitor these health promotion indicators. The variety of issues covered in the surveys included smoking prevalence and giving up smoking, alcohol consumption and knowledge about recommended drinking limits, healthier diets and eating habits, drug use and attitudes, attitudes toward contraception and sexual behaviour, sunburn and skin care in the sun (Office for National Statistics 1996).

Gender differences were found to exist in knowledge, attitudes and behaviour relating to these health promotion indicators. Men were found to be more likely than women to:

- drink more than 21 units of alcohol per week
- have taken drugs
- have had two or more sexual partners in the last year
- have been sunburnt in the last year.

However, similar proportions of men and women were current smokers.

Paradoxically, as well as being less likely to take part in risk behaviours, women were more likely to take part in behaviour which was good for their health. They were also found to be more likely than men to:

- eat low-fat varieties of food
- eat three types of starchy carbohydrates daily
- take more care in the sun.

The report states that 'the only area where men were more likely than women to engage in health behaviour was physical activity and vigorous exercise'. The report highlighted gender differences in behaviour, particularly regarding safe sex: 'a higher proportion of women than men said they would always use a condom with a new partner, although women were more likely to say they would find it difficult to raise the subject of using a condom with a new partner'. While the report highlighted the existence of behavioural differences it went on to note that attitudes were broadly the same, in that 'similar proportions of men and women said they would like to: give up smoking; drink less alcohol; take more exercise; stop using drugs' (Office for National Statistics 1996, p. 73).

Specific services

There has been increasing public interest in the need to address the health promotion needs of women and men through the provision of gender specific services, for example women's health initiatives. Generally women are in better health than they were in previous generations. Developments in health services towards improving the quality of patient care have contributed to a particular emphasis on women's

health and the provision of appropriate services. The public perception of women-centred services has usually included maternity and child care facilities. However, all aspects of reproductive health should be included, such as fertility clinics, health screening, contraception and advice services, parenting, health education and promotion. Securing the future of women- and men-specific care in a changing health care environment means that health and social care professionals will have to work together to provide an integrated, comprehensive service.

Activities

- Discuss how antenatal and postnatal services have contributed to improving public health.
- There is a trend to encourage couples to attend pre-conceptual clinics; carry out a review of the literature on this topic and discuss with your colleagues the usefulness of such a service.
- List ten good reasons why 'well-men' clinics are a valuable service.

EMPLOYMENT AND GENDER

Before the 20th century the pre-industrial economic unit of production was the household and labour tasks were divided by age and sex. With industrialisation, larger units of production were formed with people going out to work, separating home and work. This period saw the strengthening of the popular perception of paid work as masculine, particularly as more women from more affluent backgrounds were withdrawn into the separate sphere of home and family life.

Things have changed considerably since this time in that men and women exhibit different patterns of economic activity. Throughout the 20th century there has been an increase in the percentage of women in the paid workforce. In 1971 women made up 38% of the labour force compared with 44% in 1996. In spring 1996 there were almost 28 million people in the labour force in Great Britain (Central Statistics Office 1996). At this time nearly three quarters (71%)

of women of working age in the United Kingdom were economically active compared with 85% of men of working age in the UK. Although men are still more likely than women to be economically active at all ages, the gap has closed in the last 25 years. In particular the increase of women aged between 25 and 54 participating in employment can be explained by the tendency for women to give birth at an older age and then to return more quickly to the labour force. Men are also far more likely to be self-employed than women. Nearly three times more men than women are self-employed. A fundamental change in the labour market has been in the increase in the number of women employed on a part-time basis. While only 8% of male employees were working part-time, just under half (45%) of female employees were working part-time. Therefore more than five times as many women as men were part-time employees.

Paid work and occupations

After completing their initial education, most individuals enter the labour market and stay there for a significant proportion of their lives. The type of work that people do and the composition of the labour force has undergone fundamental changes in recent years. A key trend has been in the increase in the numbers of women in paid employment, particularly part-time work, and in numbers returning to work after having children. However, despite changing patterns of employment, attitudes towards women and work remain strong. The 1994 British Social Attitudes Survey, carried out by Social and Community Planning Research, asked women about their attitude to working mothers. In answer to the question 'should a woman work outside the house when her children are under school age', 55% said that she should not while 28% said that she should work part-time only; 5% said that she should work full-time.

Segregation

Attitudes towards appropriate work can affect participation in the labour force and prevalence of one gender in a particular occupation can strengthen the belief that it is particularly suited to one gender. Sex segregation is visible within the employment structure. 'Horizontal segregation' describes the distribution of men and women across different employment sectors, for example women being predominant in jobs in the service sector, the health service, teaching, and clerical and cleaning posts. In manufacturing women are concentrated in particular industries, for example footwear and clothing, food and drink, and electronic engineering assembly. 'Vertical segregation' describes the distribution of men and women in job hierarchies where men tend to have higher paid and higher status jobs than women in every sector. This draws on the view that women are less likely to be promoted at work, even when qualifications and experience are the same as men; and that job opportunities are in general worse for women than job opportunities for men with similar education and background.

A family-based explanation for gender differences in employment implies women's role as wives and mothers is primary and any paid work undertaken by women is secondary and is organised to fit in with domestic commitments. Many state services have been based on these assumptions of family functions, particularly social services. An assumption was made that a woman's wage was a second wage for the household and therefore secondary to a male wage. This family-based view does not question the sexual division of labour within a household or why women from particular social classes continue to withdraw from the labour force. A second explanation for the gendered opportunities for work centres around women as a reserve pool of labour to be drawn on as the economy demands, for example during times of war and economic expansion. The notion of a pool assumes that women and men can substitute for each other in the workforce. However, in practice, occupational segregation can be established in some occupational groups and simple substitution is rarely seen as a long term employment option by many.

Occupational segregation and associations with, for example, lower pay are often explained as 'appropriate' jobs based on skills and attributes. Often this implies biological difference and women's affinity to domestic tasks, such as caring. Dominant views on appropriate occupational segregation do put value constraints on what women and men are perceived to be able to do in the sphere of work. 'Work' may be seen to have a wider definition than paid work, and can include everything necessary to sustain life. It can be argued that feminist campaigning and knowledge have achieved to some notable extent the aim of raising the profile of unpaid caring work, and putting the idea of the unpaid career forward.

Studies of women's employment and family circumstances over the life cycle have done much to clarify patterns of gender inequality. The consideration of work histories and of the household can contribute to our understanding of gender and stratification. There is a tendency for occupations and labour processes to be sex-typed. Table 6.1 shows attitudes in the UK towards a variety of occupations and whether each occupation is seen as particularly suitable for men or for women, or for both equally. Despite many respondents to the British Social Attitudes survey indicating that in their view many of the occupations were suitable for both men and women equally, some occupations were identified as particularly suited to one gender (Social and Community Planning Research

1992). Occupations such as police officer, car mechanic, bus driver and bank manager were seen as particularly suitable for men by many respondents, while occupations such as social work, secretary and nurse were seen as particularly suitable for women.

Activity

Discuss with your colleagues whether or not you feel job categorisation still exists in British society.

HEALTH CARE A GENDERED OCCUPATION?

There are specific occupations in health care that are often viewed as suitable careers for women as they are seen as extensions of the caring role women are expected to take in society as mother, wives, daughters and so on. As an example, nursing is seen by many as caring work and to be particularly suitable for women (see Table 6.1).

It has been argued that because nursing is seen as a female dominated occupation, this has prevented it from gaining full professional status on a par with other health professions such as medicine and pharmacy. Patterns of employment confirm female dominated or sex-segregated work within the professions. While the number of men in nursing is slowly in-

Table 6.1 Gender stereotyping of occupations from British Social Attitudes Survey (Social and Community Planning Research 1992)

	Particularly suitable for men (%)	Particularly suitable for women (%)	Suitable for both equally (%)
Social work	1.0	15.0	83.1
Police officer	36.5	0.5	62.4
Secretary	0.6	54.1	44.3
Car mechanic	67.3	0.6	31.0
Nurse	0.4	31.4	67.3
Computer programmer	3.9	1.9	93.0
Bus driver	40.0	0.5	58.5
Bank manager	28.2	0.6	70.2
Family doctor/GP	5.7	0.8	92.5
Local councillor	7.2	0.9	91.0
Member of Parliament	9.6	0.5	89.2

Table 6.2   Gender Analysis of the UKCC Effective Register by part of the register, 1995 from UKCC Statistical Analysis of the Council's Professional Register, 1 April 1995 to 31 March 1996 (December 1996)

Part of the register	Male (%)	Female (%)
Part 1: First level nurses trained in general nursing	5.84	94.16
Part 2: Second level nurses trained in general nursing (England & Wales)	4.18	95.82
Part 3: First level nurses trained in the nursing of persons suffering from mental illness	39.16	60.84
Part 4: Second level nurses trained in the nursing of persons suffering from mental illness (England & Wales)	27.66	72.34
Part 5: First level nurses trained in the nursing of persons suffering from mental handicap	35.83	64.17
Part 6: Second level nurses trained in the nursing of persons suffering from mental handicap (England & Wales)	27.43	72.57
Part 7: Second level nurses (Scotland & Northern Ireland)	8.35	91.65
Part 8: Nurses trained in the nursing of sick children	2.30	97.70
Part 9: Nurses trained in the nursing of persons suffering from fever	1.29	98.71
Part 10: Midwives	0.14	99.86
Part 11: Health visitors	1.06	98.94
Part 12: First level nurses trained in adult nursing*	8.98	91.02
Part 13: First level nurses trained in mental health nursing*	33.74	66.26
Part 14: First level nurses trained in mental handicap nursing*	25.64	74.36
Part 15: First level nurses trained in children's nursing*	5.73	94.27

*Project 2000 courses

creasing (from 8.3% of those on the effective register[1] in 1990 to 9.2% in 1996 (UKCC 1996)), nursing is still a female dominated occupation. Nine out of ten registered nurses on the effective register are women. However, although a female dominated profession, gender stratification may be seen within nursing. Table 6.2 shows a gender analysis of parts of the UKCC register which correspond to different nursing qualifications.

While women predominate in general nursing, midwifery, health visiting and children's nursing, men are far more likely to work in mental health nursing and learning disabilities (mental handicap) nursing. Vertical segregation is also visible from examining employment patterns in nursing with men in nursing often progressing at a quicker rate than women up the career ladder, holding more senior positions, and different career progressions. A contributory factor to this pattern is that while many women have an inter-

rupted career pattern because of maternity leave and caring responsibilities, in contrast many men have patterns of continuous paid employment.

Activities

- List ten reasons why you think 91% of nurses are women.
- Organise a debate to discuss the role of men in nursing.

Gender and informal care

Distinctions have been suggested between informal and formal care. Davies (1995) proposes a distinction between care giving, care work and professional care.

Women play a crucial role in the health of the nation as carers and providers for their families (RCN 1992). Culturally women are associated with providing informal care, and this view can be seen to influence the perceptions of many caring professions as suitable jobs for women. For many women their pattern of paid work

[1] The United Kingdom Central Council for Nursing, Midwifery and Health Visiting is the regulatory body for the nursing, midwifery and health visiting professions throughout the UK. Registered nurses, midwives and health visitors are required to hold effective registration with the UKCC if they wish to practise.

may be influenced by domestic commitments. Indeed, as the following discussion focusing on registered nurses demonstrates, work patterns may have to change to cater for those caring at home as well as during paid employment. Nursing is a 'caring' profession, but many individual nurses also have caring responsibilities outside work, which can affect their availability for paid employment.

Demographic changes

Demographic change and labour market trends suggest that employers will have to take greater account of their employees' caring responsibilities over the next few years. Women have accounted for much of the growth in the labour force since the mid-1980s. As the impact of the recession has been concentrated amongst men and full-timers, there are now parts of the country where there are more women employed than men (Income Data Services 1993). This pattern is expected to continue, with women accounting for over 80% of the labour force growth, and 46% of the labour force in the next decade. By 2001 there will be a greater proportion of older workers and women in employment in the UK labour force. Labour force growth is projected to occur predominantly in the older age groups. During the next 10 years those aged 35 and over are expected to increase by almost 3 million (19%), with specific expansion in the number of people employed aged between 45 and 54 years. Nursing is mirroring this trend – the average age of nurses on the UKCC register is increasing.

Older people

Today, all over the world, older people are the main consumers of health, social services and nursing care. Many older people can expect to enjoy a healthy old age, but the proportion of the very oldest who are frail and potentially vulnerable will increase. These older people will increasingly require more time, more money, more resources and more people to look after them. In future, growing numbers of older people will be cared for in their own homes, or in residential or nursing homes as well as in the hospital. Hospital care for older people is also changing as more hospitals are merging services for older people with acute medicine as the number of older people needing hospital care increases.

By 2021 more than 30% of the UK population will be between 50 and 74 – i.e. 19 million people will require social services, pensions and, above all, care. Much of the direct care and support for older people in the hospital setting will be provided by nurses. Some of the most innovative nursing work is taking place in the care of older people. However, the majority of that care provided to older people will be by an unpaid group of relatives and friends, mainly women, many of whom juggle their caring role with paid employment.

Informal caring

The campaigning group Caring Costs has estimated that informal caring saves the country up to £24 billion each year in wages (Pilkington 1993). Many employers have so far failed to identify the scale of caring being carried out by employees. Recent studies have shown that the caring responsibilities of nurses have a significant bearing on their availability to work, on their career planning and on their mobility (Seccombe and Ball 1992). Those who care for dependants fall into two distinct age groups. Nearly one third of a sample of 4000 nurses aged between 26 and 35 had children of pre-school age while nearly a quarter of those in the 46–55 age group and a fifth aged 56 and over cared for dependent adults. (Seccombe & Ball 1992). This suggests that the caring role is often unbroken for many who, having spent years looking after their children, find themselves with the responsibility of caring for an older relative or a sick partner. The majority of nurses view hours fitting in with social and domestic circumstances as very important. More than a third rate hours fitting in with social and domestic circumstances as the most important work related factor (Buchan and Seccombe 1991).

While only a small proportion of carers give up work to care for their dependants, many change their working patterns in some way. Many lose time from work or have to take time off, resulting in increased absence rates. Others take a reduction in working hours from full-time to part-time employment, or change their hours to best suit their other commitments. Survey evidence has shown that those caring for dependent adults, with no dependent children, are nearly twice as likely to be working part-time as those with no dependants (Seccombe & Ball 1992). More than one in five reported that caring for a dependent adult affected their ability to work. Overall just over half had caring responsibilities for either dependent children or adults, with over one in ten having responsibility for dependent children and adults.

The ageing workforce and population have important implications for patterns of work, the demand for job-share posts, part-time work and flexible working, and also for career opportunities and post-registration training for mature nurses. The Carnegie Inquiry into the Third Age recommended that employers should help staff caring for dependants through schemes such as part-time working and paid leave (Carnegie UK Trust 1993). The introduction of flexible working can ease the stress of juggling work and caring responsibilities. The most common route some employers in the private sector have taken to help their employees who care for dependent adults is extending existing career break schemes. Another is helpline services providing advice, counselling and referrals to other agencies for further help.

While more advanced arrangements such as support groups, referral services and adult day care are beginning to appear in the USA, in the UK the care of older dependants is just beginning to be recognised as an issue. The care of older people is mainly thought of as a family concern or the responsibility of the state. However, policies such as care in the community and demographic changes of an ageing population and more women entering the workforce will eventually force the issue onto employers' agendas.

While distinctions may be made between informal and formal care, it has been argued that policy developments in the United Kingdom are breaking down the boundaries between formal and informal care (Ungerson 1995). Indeed where payment for care is concerned, Ungerson (1995) argues that the blurring of boundaries is particularly evident and that 'benefits systems are actually a form of commodification of the caring relationship' with potential results for the relationship between the person giving the care and the person receiving care.

Activities

- Consider with your colleagues why caring for dependent relatives in the home remains the responsibility of women.
- Outline what you think the government could do to relieve the burden of informal care, particularly in terms of distributing the responsibility of providing care among male family members.

SELF-AWARENESS OF BELIEFS AND PRACTICES

Whichever theory of gender relations most closely matches your own views, it is beneficial to examine your attitudes and beliefs. Consider how they affect your perceptions of men and women and how this might influence the care you provide as a health care professional. The discussions outlined above on health chances, the labour market, gendered occupations and informal care provide examples of areas to consider.

This chapter has identified some of the factors which can affect men's and women's experience of health and illness, and has explored the complex relationships between gender issues and health. Theories of gender have been examined with analysis of different approaches to understanding gender divisions, including feminist approaches. Consideration has been given to gender and inequality in health care including issues of health chances and health promotion activity with specific targeted health services for men and women. In addition health work as a gendered occupation has been considered within the context of the UK labour force, paid work and informal care. Finally, you have been asked to consider your awareness of your own beliefs and practices towards gender issues.

Meeting the health needs of women and men requires that health professionals not only communicate effectively with patients, but that they collaborate with each other to understand the whole range of physical and emotional needs of sick and well individuals. The approach to day-to-day care must take account of differences in perceptions about women and men to ensure that appropriate care is provided as needed. To provide quality health services aimed specifically for women or men on particular health issues, the complete emotional and physical

well-being must be catered for and not simply the condition for which treatment or care is required. Essential links must be forged between hospital services and other NHS primary and community services. Care must be patient centred so that the individual and their carers experience an integrated health system.

Activities

- Carry out a review of the literature on the subject of gender and health care.
- Discuss with your colleagues evidence of inequality or gender division.
- Having worked through this chapter, discuss with your colleagues how you feel about the issue of gender as an issue of social policy and health care.

REFERENCES

Brownmillar S 1975 Against Our Will: Men, Women and Rape. Secker and Warburg, London

Buchan J, Seccombe I 1991 Nurses' work and worth. IMS Report No 213. Institute of Manpower Studies, Brighton

Carnegie United Kingdom Trust 1993 Life, work and livelihood in the third age. April. Carnegie UKT, Dunfermline

Collier J, Rosaldo M 1981 Politics and gender in simple societies. In Ortner S, Whitehead H (eds) Sexual Meanings. Cambridge University Press, Cambridge

Dalla Costa M, James S 1975 The power of women and the subversion of the community, 3rd edn. Falling Wall Press, Bristol

Davies C 1995 Competence versus care: gender and caring work revisited. Acta-Sociologica 38(1): 17–31

Delphy C 1984 Close to home: a materialist analysis of women's oppression. Hutchison in association with Explorations in Feminism Collection, London

Eisenstein Z 1979 Developing a theory of capitalist patriarchy and socialist feminism. In Eisenstein Z (ed) 1979 Capitalist patriarchy and the case for socialist feminism. Monthly Review Press, London

Engels F 1986 The origin of the family, private property and the state. Penguin, Harmondsworth

Firestone S 1979 The dialectic of sex: the case for feminist revolution. Women's Press, London

Graham H 1995 Gender and class as dimensions of smoking behaviour in Britain: insights from a survey of mothers. Social Science and Medicine 38(5):691–698

Hartmann H 1981 The unhappy marriage of Marxism and feminism: towards a more progressive union. In Sargent L (ed) 1981 Women and revolution: a discussion of the unhappy marriage of Marxism and feminism. Pluto, London

Income Data Services 1993 Report 640 IDS, London

Millett K 1971 Sexual politics. Hart–Davis, London

Mitchell J 1971 Women's estate. Penguin, Harmondsworth

Moore H 1988 Feminism and anthropology. Polity, Cambridge

Office for National Statistics 1996 Health in England: what people know, what people think, what people do. The Stationery Office, London

Office for National Statistics 1995 Social Trends 25. The Stationery Office, London

Office for National Statistics 1996 Social Trends 26. The Stationery Office, London

Office for National Statistics 1997 Social Trends 27. The Stationery Office, London

Office for National Statistics Social Survey Division 1997 Living in Britain: results from the 1995 General Household Survey. HMSO, London

Office of Population Censuses and Surveys Social Survey Division 1996 Living in Britain: results from the 1994 General Household Survey. HMSO, London

Parsons T 1955 Family, socialization and interaction process. Free Press, London

Pilkington E 1993 Speech was like a feminist testament from the 1970s. The Guardian (Wednesday 2 June, p. 20)

Royal College of Nursing 1992 Health of half the nation. RCN, London

United Kingdom Central Council 1996 Statistical analysis of the council's professional register, 1 April 1995 to 31 March 1996. UKCC, London

Seccombe I, Ball J 1992 Motivation, morale and mobility. IMS Report No. 233. Institute of Manpower Studies, Brighton

Social and Community Planning Research 1992 British social attitudes cumulative sourcebook: the first six surveys. Gower, Aldershot

Social and Community Planning Research 1994 British social attitudes. Gower, Aldershot

Ungerson C 1995 Gender, cash and informal care: European perspectives and dilemmas. Journal of Social Policy 24(1 Jan):31–52

Wilkinson S, Kitzinger C (eds) 1994 Women and health: feminist perspectives. Taylor & Francis, London

Williams F 1989 Social policy: a critical introduction: issues of race, gender and class. Polity Press, Cambridge

Women and Geography Study Group 1984 Geography and gender: an introduction to feminist geography. Hutchinson, London

Zaretsky E 1976 Capitalism, the family and personal life. Pluto Press, London

2

Focal issues

The Welfare Sate, which the Government introduced after the Second World War, provided a framework for meeting the essential and fundamental objectives of a fair and just health and social service that is equally and equitably distributed. From this premise the chapters in this section consider government attempts to meet the twin objectives of providing quality services and, at the same time, control public spending. This section will also provide an examination of discrete policies and services for specific client groups.

Reorganised health care

Kevin Gormley

After studying this chapter the student should be able to:

- **highlight the emerging difficulties with providing a universal health care system**
- **describe the reasons why changes in management and reorganisation of the NHS were necessary**
- **discuss the measures that were initiated by government to meet the changing health care needs of society**
- **appreciate the process of implementing phased change in health care provision towards an overall objective**

Introduction

This chapter will build on the contents of previous chapters which addressed issues such as the origins of welfare and the NHS. It will examine the key influences on the health service, particularly as reorganisation became a major factor. Considerable attention will be paid to the economic and political climate that existed as these changes were enacted. The chapter will go on to provide some of the reasoning of the new right which in many ways marked the return of the classical utilitarian doctrine of the last century. Contrasts will then be drawn between the political consensus that originally existed and was characterised by a balance between market-based philosophies and state intervention, and the present.

THE EARLY IDEAS

The NHS that Aneurin Bevan introduced in 1948 was underlined by two clear principles. First it would be an equal and equitable service that would be free at the point of use. This principle ensured that the sick would not have to pay for their care at a time when they were most vulnerable and the amount of contributions made had no bearing on how much care they would receive. The 'free at the point of use' principle was tested as early as 1949 when Bevan introduced a nominal charge for medical prescriptions. Although the reason for its introduction was financially sound in that it prevented a limitation on health service spending, the early principle of free at the point of use was compromised.

The second principle was the commitment to eliminating the backlog of ill-health that existed at the time. To this end Bevan continued to introduce costly expenditure programmes to the NHS in the belief that a modernised service would quicken the anticipated fall in demand for services. Once again this ideal proved difficult to achieve. As hospitals grew in size and the range and complexity of services extended, it soon became clear that new problems were replacing those that the service was originally designed to resolve. Health care, it seemed, was like an advanced form of Parkinson's law: any increase in provision was met by a corresponding increase in demand (Ham 1985, 1991).

EVALUATION OF THE SERVICE – THE BEGINNING OF CHANGE

The introduction of the NHS was a radical change and needed time to bed down before any worthwhile evaluation of the service could be made. The service was also held in very high esteem among the general public. For these reasons it was difficult for the government to consider any serious change, even if it wanted to. Although additional charges were introduced for dentures and spectacles the structure and function of the NHS changed very little in its early days.

The first significant economic test on the NHS was the substantive rise in costs of the pharma-ceutical industry. Early planners of the NHS had not considered the fact that new compounds had been discovered that were now assisting in the treatment of hypertension, diabetes, mental illness, infectious disease and cancer. Additionally, new anaesthetic agents facilitated advanced and expensive surgical methods which could now be undertaken more safely. The Guillebaud Report, which examined health care spending, informed the government that proportionate to the gross national product, the actual cost of the health service had fallen from 3.75% in 1949 to 3.25% in 1954 and that there were no grounds for suggesting any excessive extravagance in the service (Guillebaud Committee 1956). Politicians were, however, uneasy about the seemingly open-ended management structure and lack of accountability.

The criticism of management was blamed on the excessive clinical freedom and influence exerted by the medical profession. This was not totally unexpected given the unique organisational arrangements that existed. On the one hand the medical profession controlled the demand for financial resources from central government. On the other hand they were also accountable for its distribution and spending. The Bradbeer Committee (Central Health Services Council 1954) commented that the custom of appointing a medical representative as hospital secretary was unnecessary and wasteful. It was argued that the control of financial arrangements and the management of hospital administrative, catering and ancillary staff should be managed by separate managerial arrangements. The committee proposed the appointment of an administrative representative on hospital management committees and that this indivi-

Activities

- List five reasons why you think the medical profession was a particularly dominant group in the early days of the NHS.
- Why was it considered unnecessary for the hospital secretary to be a doctor?

dual should not have either a medical or nursing background. These proposals were, in time, accepted and new arrangements were initiated that created a career structure for hospital administrators in terms of grading, recruitment, training and promotion (Owen 1988).

A need for managerial and organisational change

Managerial

By the 1960s it became more clear that there was a need for change in the administrative structure of the NHS. The Porritt Report (Medical Services Review Committee 1962), which was compiled independent of the Ministry of Health by representatives of the medical profession, called for a substantial overhaul of the management structure of the NHS. Around the same time, the Minister of Health, Enoch Powell, proposed a major hospital building plan but in the same report identified a need to reappraise the existing structures for managing the hospital services (Advisory Committee 1966, Ministry of Health 1962).

Two reports were later published, each of which contained proposals that were quite different. The Farquharson-Lang Committee (Scottish Health Services Council 1966) was set up to examine administrative structures in Scotland that could have implications for the remainder of the United Kingdom. It proposed the appointment of a chief executive to each of Scotland's boards who would be accountable for services as well as regulating and commissioning new capital projects. The proposals contained in this report were not accepted, probably because the same year the larger and more influential Salmon Committee had reported to the Ministry with suggestions for a new senior nurse management structure for nurses (Ministry of Health 1966). The Salmon Committee contended that the contribution made by senior nurses to the service had not been recognised, particularly in terms of authority, status or influence in decision making. To redress this issue the committee recommended consensus managerial arrangements rather than individual decision making,

which was in contrast to the Scottish template. It was proposed that a chief nursing officer should be appointed in an executive position within each regional health authority and reciprocal appointments should be made at district and local level. The Salmon Report was accepted by the secretary of state and introduced on a pilot basis from 1967–72 (Harrison 1988, Levitt et al 1995).

Activities

- Discuss with your colleagues whether final decisions are best made by one individual or by a group of experts.
- Do you feel it was right to involve nurses in major health care decisions?

REORGANISATION

The new Conservative government of 1970 continued the process of reorganisation that had been started by Richard Crossman but with more vigour. The secretary of state, Sir Keith Joseph, commissioned a team of outside business advisers to investigate the administration of the service before publishing a new White Paper (DHSS 1972a). This publication was broadly similar to the Green Paper published by his predecessor. A further publication in the same year, referred to as the Grey Book (DHSS 1972b) detailed precisely the new arrangements (see Box 7.1).

The 1973 NHS Reorganisation Act was introduced coincidentally on 5 July of that year, 25 years to the day after the introduction of the National Health Service. In spite of opposing many of the changes while in opposition, the incoming Labour government adhered to the previous Conservative legislation. The only amendment to the Act was an increase in the number of local government representatives on health authorities. This was important because it did at least give some measure of public accountability, given that the remainder of members on the new authorities were appointees. This amend-

---

Box 7.1 First reorganisation

The main changes were as follows:

- a new structure of regional health authorities, area health authorities and district management teams
- the disappearance of the special position of teaching hospitals
- the amalgamation of hospital with community services
- the separate administrative arrangements for GPs would be retained but would now be called family practitioner committees and would operate under the direct control of the new area health authorities
- community health professionals, including health visitors and district nurses, would form new primary care teams
- all senior staff undertake in-service management training in order to fully appreciate and implement the new management philosophy of consensus management and specialisation

---

Box 7.2 New management functions

- 14 regional health authorities were directly responsible to the DHSS. They adopted responsibility for strategic planning, capital spending and the provision of services.
- Below this tier, 90 area health authorities were created, most of which were further sub-divided into districts. There were 205 districts in England and Wales, each representing a population of around 200,000 people.
- Area health authorities were accountable for assessing precise need in terms of both hospital and community services as well as the day-to-day provision of services. They were forced to exercise economic restraint because finite limits of money were allocated to them. Any proposed service that potentially incurred additional funding was rigorously scrutinised by the regional body.

---

ment was also in keeping with the proposals in the earlier Green Paper (Lister 1988, Ranade 1994).

Reasons for reorganisation

Distribution of services

The government's aim in reorganisation was to try and achieve equity in the distribution of services. It had previously been assumed that a fair level of health care facilities could be provided simply by measuring the extent of need and then providing that service. Under the new structure additional services had to be considered in terms of the availability of resources and the potential for the discontinuation of other services which were either no longer necessary or not essential. Reorganisation was also a way of introducing balance in the funding between the centrally controlled hospital and local authority personal and social services. In line with this aim the management structure and function was significantly changed (see Box 7.2). The principle of consensus management was also safeguarded in that agreement had to be reached between committee members before decisions could be passed up or down to the appropriate tier of decision making (Baggott 1994, Klein 1989, Owen 1988).

 Activities

Discuss with your colleagues:

- the reasons why it was necessary to reorganise the NHS
- whether or not these changes improved the service to patients.

FURTHER REFORM

Economic crisis

In spite of the changes discontent remained. The world economic crisis during this period, precipitated partly by the spiralling increase in the price of oil, resulted in generally poor economic performance in many developing nations. This exacerbated the heavy burden of debt on many countries, including Britain. As a result Britain had to undergo a process of economic stabilisation alongside further structural adjustments. This caused a devaluation of currency which produced a reduction in the ability of government to meet even existing public spending requirements and an increase in the retail price of goods. Given this difficult economic situation, the government had to implement firmer financial control of the money allotted to regional authorities. The economic crisis also lowered the value of wages, including those of health care staff. The general public were also dissatisfied because high inflation limited area health authorities' ability to provide existing services, let alone continue to meet the demand for expansion. The net effect, at least in the public's perception, was a poorer quality of service and longer waiting times for operations.

The cost of providing a national health service, as mentioned earlier in the chapter, has always been a political issue, but never more so than in the 1970s. It was estimated that spending on health care in 1953 was approximately £433 million. By the mid-1970s the cost had risen to £6879 million per annum. Costs had risen in all sectors of the service but the rise was particularly significant in the acute hospital sector. The rise in costs can be attributed to expensive technological innovation along with growing expectation and aspirations by health care professionals and patients. For example, in the mid-1950s the standard treatment for osteoarthritis of the hip would have been pain-relieving medication, physiotherapy and a recommendation by the doctor that the patient should change her lifestyle in order to adjust to a life of dependence and impaired mobility. This programme of care was almost totally replaced by surgical intervention, with hip replacements becoming the normally expected plan for dealing with this problem. It was therefore necessary that new aims in keeping with new trends in health care should be produced (Able-Smith 1994, Owen 1988).

Activities

* List five reasons which caused the economic crisis of the 1970s.
* Consider why this may have affected health care provision.

The Royal Commission on the National Health Service

Only a few years after the first major reorganisa-

Box 7.3 The Merrison Report

The Merrison Report investigation included:

* the allocation of resources to less affluent areas
* the care of vulnerable groups such as the old and the mentally ill
* the level of collaboration between health and social services staff
* poor industrial relations within the NHS

tion, and in an attempt to quell public discontent, the prime minister, Harold Wilson, announced he was to set up a Royal Commission under the chairmanship of Sir Alec Merrison. The Commission was asked to address a number of key issues in the health service (see Box 7.3).

The report of the Royal Commission was published in 1979 (Cmnd 7615). In some ways it reiterated many of the principles espoused by Bevan, in that it reaffirmed the need for the service to be equitably distributed, reflecting fairness in the service. The Commission also agreed that health care should continue to be free at the point of use but added that the service should also have a greater emphasis on promoting health and preventing the incidence of disease. It went on, however, to indicate some of the changes that were required and which did eventually come about in the 1980s. Most pertinent, the Commission admitted that the NHS could not meet all the public demands for health care. To this end it accepted that managerial choices had to be made at all levels of the service as to where need would and would not be met (Harrison 1988).

Patients First

Following the election of Margaret Thatcher as prime minister, the speed and extent of health care reform increased. The government was ideologically influenced by the academic argument of the new right, a group within the Conservative party which espoused the value of the free-market principle and the privatisation of state monopolised industries; it also called for a restructuring of the system of welfare provision, particularly the NHS. The government began the process by first of all discarding the Health Service Board which had been initially set up to monitor and regulate the growth of the private sector. The previous policy of phasing out pay beds was reversed and consultants were permitted to earn up to 10% of their salary outside the NHS without incurring any deductions in their full-time pay.

More important, the government quickly introduced another round of restructuring with the publication of the consultative document, *Patients First* (DHSS 1979). This publication recommended the gradual replacement of area health authorities with a firmer managerial district tier of organisation. This would leave the power and control of services with regional authorities but devolve the day-to-day running of services and local decision making as near to the point of delivery as possible (Ranade 1994).

Activity

The Royal Commission of 1979 recognised that the NHS could not keep pace with the public demand for services. With your colleagues select any two different areas of health care provision (such as maternity services, care of the elderly, mental health, surgery) and organise a debate to discuss which of them should be given priority. Then discuss your conclusions.

General management

The implementation of change was impeded by the consensus management system that had been introduced in 1974. It was argued that consensus management made it almost impossible to achieve full agreement, thereby slowing down any decision making. Sir Roy Griffith, the managing director of Sainsbury's, was appointed to advise the minister as to the best way of resolving this difficulty. Griffith suggested to the secretary of state that the difficulty could be resolved through the appointment of general managers at every level of the NHS organisation (DHSS 1983). Griffith proposed that general managers should be appointed on fixed term contracts with a remit to improve efficiency. This

would probably be achieved through implementing difficult and unpopular policies such as the contracting-out of services. The following year the secretary of state announced that he had accepted the idea and subsequently issued a circular (DHSS 1984) directing general manager appointments. Soon afterwards managers were appointed at all levels and spheres of the service, including mental health, general hospitals, community services, care of the elderly services, domestic services and so on. Each local or service general manager reported to the district general manager, who in turn reported directly to the regional general manager.

As the system settled, general manager training programmes were set in place for the effective preparation of people who wished to pursue a career in health service management. The product of these management preparation programmes created three distinct categories of manager. First there were first line managers who for the most part worked in a supervisory role. Second there were middle managers who were operational heads of departments but not necessarily from a specific professional group. Third there were senior managers who were few in number but centrally situated and whose main role was strategic planning (James 1994, Levitt et al 1995).

Activity

Organise a visit from one of your local general managers to discuss the role and responsibility of the position and its relationship with health care professions.

Business solution

The key factor in this policy was that it enabled the imposition of a business solution to the spiralling costs of health care provision. The form of business solution that eventually emerged was essentially fourfold (see Box 7.4).

The introduction of general managers assured the government that a clear and effective chain

Box 7.4 Business solution to spiralling costs in health care

- wherever possible the dictate of the market should make decisions about health and welfare spending
- if stimulated properly the private sector organisations could be more effective than public sector services
- financial accountability should take precedence over all other considerations
- business decisions should be rational and management driven (James 1994)

Box 7.5 New strategies for efficiency and accountability

- resource management
- performance indicators
- performance review
- auditing of services
- communication
- management development

of command was in place from the point of delivery all the way up to the NHS management executive and the secretary of state (DHSS 1989). In changing the managerial arrangements of the NHS, the government was also able to implement a series of new strategies which reinforced the objectives of efficiency and accountability (see Box 7.5). Each of these was designed to put the health service on a business footing.

Activities

- List the differences that the introduction of general managers made in terms of administering the health service.
- Organise a debate with your colleagues to discuss whether or not the introduction of general managers at this time was appropriate.

DECENTRALISATION

When the *Patients First* document was introduced it was accepted that it was also a programme for decentralisation. Decentralisation

in health policy terms meant the transfer of resources for planning, managing and the generation and allocation of resources from the control of central government and its associated agencies to the lowest possible line of management. In the longer term this would mean a self-governing authority or trust. Politicians who supported the idea of decentralised health care services argued that it was a perfect vehicle for increasing the participation of the community in decision making. They also contended that it ensured that services were appropriate for a given population and that they reflected actual need and were patient led. Opponents of this view suggest that it diluted the NHS and made it even more difficult to sustain the principles of equality, equity and universalism (Gormley 1996).

MONEY IN HEALTH CARE

From the early 1980s the government introduced a range of measures that made the movement of money more obvious in health care (Box 7.6 and Box 7.7). While this did provide a quantitative measure of efficiency it was only successful so long as it was transparent that the ethos of a free service remained.

Money allocated to health authorities can be spent in different ways. At a simple or traditional level it can be used to provide statutory services. Alternatively the money could be used for contracting outside services if they are judged to be cheaper and more efficient. To prevent any reduction in quality of services, time limited contracts are negotiated. Money is also used to promote health policies such as breast or cervical

Box 7.6 Increasing the influence of money

The purpose of increasing the influence of money was to:

- open up a health care market
- introduce an element of competition for services
- allow for an element of choice on the part of purchasers of care
- create a higher profile of managerialism and accountability at every level of the service

Box 7.7 Money and the NHS

Introduction of money and the NHS

- *Fee for service*: itemising through internal audit a cost factor on each individual service such as paramedical expertise (physiotherapy or speech therapy) or products such as specific pharmaceuticals. In carrying out this process a measurement is provided which allows for the accurate recording of increases in efficiency or financial savings.
- *Case payment*: in this situation a total package of care is costed by an independent/brokerage system. A care manager working within a fixed budget has a responsibility to meet the needs of patients but at the same time remain within the total budgetary allocation. This is frequently used as a mechanism for organising services in the community.
- *Capitation*: this is a system used by general practitioners. A fixed payment is allowed by a local authority for each person on a practice's list. As an incentive to have a mixed case load of patients, additional allowances are allocated for certain population groups such as a given number of people over 75 years of age.
- *Global funding*: this is the budgetary allowance usually provided to trusts. It is an all inclusive operating figure set out at the beginning of the year and provides a ceiling for spending, but at the same time allows for flexibility in the allocation of money within the limit so long as the criteria for services laid down by the purchaser (local authority/board) have been met.

(WHO 1993)

screening or to stimulate an alternative provider of a service, such as the private or voluntary sector. Some trusts have entered into contracts with voluntary hospice associations for the provision of palliative care services.

Money can also be given directly to individuals within the service as a form of incentive to adhere to targets. General practitioners, for example, receive special bonuses if they achieve specific preventive targets such as immunisation programmes or if they invest in specific

Activity

With your colleagues:

- Consider why the government adopted a strategy of costing all services.

equipment for their practice. This payment is in addition to their salaries and capitation fees.

HEALTH CARE INTO THE 1990s

In 1990 the government introduced the NHS and Community Care Act, which outlined the strategic plans for the provision of health and social services throughout the United Kingdom. This Act was the end product of three White Papers: *Working for Patients* (Department of Health 1989a); *Caring for People* (Department of Health 1989b); and *Health Service Management Resource Assumption and Planning Guidelines* (Department of Health 1989), and was implemented over a phased 3-year period.

Working for Patients

Soon after the implementation of *Patients First*, plans were under way for the next set of proposals for further reorganisation of the service. In spite of major successes in efficiency the government still was not satisfied with the structure and organisation of the service. Work commenced on introducing changes that would place the service on a firm business footing. The eventual blueprint was released by the Secretary of State for Health, Kenneth Clarke, in a White Paper: *Working for Patients* (Dept of Health 1989).

The spectacular launch of this document was at the Limehouse Studios in London's docklands. The arrival of Mr Clarke by boat, sailing from Westminster, was reminiscent of the arrival of Grace O'Malley, the Irish pirate who, in the 16th century, had boldly sailed up the Thames in a blaze of glory to sign a peace pact with Henry VIII. On this occasion the audience was a selected group of representatives from adjacent regional health authorities who were informed by the minister that this was the most radical reform of the NHS since its inception.

Working for Patients provided guidelines for new systems of management and financial and quality control (see Box 7.8) in order to deliver goods or services more cost-effectively to patients (Dent 1995, Hancock 1995, Sines 1995).

> **Box 7.8 Working for Patients – objectives**
>
> Four clear objectives were identified in the *Working for Patients* strategy: it would:
>
> - create a system of controlling the distribution of all resources
> - involve clinicians in the management and control of budgets
> - introduce mechanisms for assessing the quality of services as well as quantitative indicators of level of services
> - provide adequate and appropriate information to permit better decision making

Resource management initiative

The proposals also contained a commitment to continuing the resource management initiative which had been launched in 1986. When *Working for Patients* was published, resource management had already created a health care system wherein all services could be costed. This in turn created the dynamic for the key proposal of *Working for Patients*, that resource management should move towards the development of an internal market. This effectively was the beginning of the contract culture within the NHS.

Working for Patients fostered the idea that money should follow patients. It was from this premise that most of the main proposals contained in the White Paper emanated; they included:

- the introduction of weighted capitation (that is the allocation of money to districts based on the numbers of people resident in the catchment area)
- there would be regular independent auditing of NHS spending
- the stimulation of a separation of functions of the health service between providing and purchasing
- the creation of NHS Trusts with the freedom to set pay levels or borrow for capital funding projects
- new controls of consultants' contracts and conditions of services
- larger GP practices would be allotted separate budgetary allowances for the purchase of a selected range of health care services.

Activity

What is meant by the term: money should follow patients?

Caring for people

The White Paper *Caring for People* (Department of Health 1989) and the resultant National Health Service and Community Care Act was the government's positive response to Sir Roy Griffith's second report (Griffith 1988). In the first instance the White Paper affirmed that all statutory services should strive towards higher levels of partnership and also to maximise co-operation with the voluntary and private sectors. This would create a seamless and comprehensive range of services for dependent people (the elderly, people with a learning disability and mental health problems).

Alongside this it was noted that new organisations within the statutory sector have each created their own elaborate managerial systems which do not complement each other. It had been suggested that this structural managerial deficit could be addressed by the appointment of a care manager (Davis & Challis 1986). This eventually became a central theme of the next round of Griffith proposals. The question as to which professional group should take on this role was also addressed in the report (Griffith 1988). However, no definitive response was provided as Griffith took the view that the imposition of a mandatory solution at that stage would only distract personnel away from concentrating on performance and accountability. *Caring for People*, however, recommended clearly that care managers should be appointed from personnel working in social services departments of local authorities.

Care management

Care managers, it was envisaged, would take on the role of facilitators, ensuring that care was provided, rather than actually providing the

> **Box 7.9 Care management**
>
> Care management encompasses a range of core skills:
>
> - case finding
> - screening
> - accurate assessment of need
> - care planning
> - monitoring
> - evaluation of services that are provided

service. Within this framework *Caring for People* reinforced the existing policy of extending the range of providers from the rapidly growing areas of the voluntary and private sectors along with the existing statutory provision. Care management in practice was designed to adopt a needs-led strategy in order to assist people who have difficulty in meeting their individual needs (see Box 7.9). In simpler terms it is a mechanism for identifying people who require attention, appreciating their particular needs, constructing a programme of care from a range of services, keeping in touch to evaluate the effectiveness of the programme and finally making appropriate adjustments as necessary (Audit Commission 1992, Davis and Challis 1986).

Activity

Why was it necessary to introducing care management into community services?

EFFECTS OF THE HEALTH SERVICE CHANGES

Government role

The change in the role and function of government has been the most evident amendment to the NHS. Whether the *raison d'être* for this is economic necessity, political conviction or a combination of both is open to debate. It is nevertheless a fact that the direct financial input by government, especially for the most vulner-

able client groups, has been superseded by private contractual arrangements. The government's role has, however, remained significant in two specific areas. First, as a policy maker, the government contributes significantly through, for example, tax concessions or subsidies to the private sector to create an economic environment conducive to the economic changes currently being implemented in the health service. Second, the government sets national health priorities and determines the mechanism through which objectives can ultimately be achieved.

In order for these roles to be fulfilled the government has also emerged as a valuable information resource through the encouragement of research and the accumulation of up-to-date and accurate population data. Information is also collated in the areas including financial distribution and the relationships between the private, voluntary and public sector services.

Activity

- How has the role of government changed in health care provision since the beginning of the NHS in 1948?
- Is this new role appropriate?

PATIENTS

During the mid-1980s, during all this change, there were also attempts to improve the rights of patients. For example patients were permitted limited access to their medical records. Additionally the *Patient's Charter* (DoH 1991a) was introduced as a mechanism to improve patient involvement and to make the service more responsive to patient needs. Excepting these improvements, the patient has remained the only player whose role has not significantly changed in the revised health service. This will probably remain the case for as long as many patients have neither the necessary knowledge nor the desire to contribute to decision making. Until this changes the power and authority to make decisions concerning the choice and selection of treatment programmes will remain the domain of the medical profession.

The potential for involving patients in health care decisions is dependent on two factors. First ensuring that the necessary information is readily available and second, allowing consumers to use this information to make their own decisions. Since paternalism formed the cornerstone of the early NHS, from the outset the general public and consumers were encouraged by government to leave matters of health care to professionals. It is at present difficult to imagine a time when patients, on a large scale, might wish to shoulder the responsibility of deciding what services should and should not be provided for them and their fellow citizens.

The only avenue currently available for patients who wish to express their views regarding the nature of health services is via the political process and the exertion of pressure groups. A notable example of this has been in the field of maternity services. As a result of pressure brought to bear by women both individually and, collectively, in support groups, substantive changes have been introduced. Women are now in a position to decide where, when and how they would prefer to have their babies delivered and by whom. In addition they now have access to a full complement of health education and promotion services before conception, antenatally and for a period after they have delivered their babies (Butler 1993).

Activity

List five reasons why patients do not take the lead in making individual health care decisions.

Summary

As the new millenium approaches, health service personnel face constant changes in the distribution of health care provision. They have already found their roles, work and traditional influencing processes challenged. In addition the demand for evidence-based health care is

putting added pressure on them to demonstrate their value to purchasers and providers of services. The problems with organising health care are effectively threefold. The first challenge is ensuring a reasonable level of resource. This is difficult, particularly in times of recession when other services such as education, defence and industry are looking for a share of the gross domestic product. The second is the problem of priorities in the distribution of resources. Given the increasingly high cost of care, as the Merrison Report highlighted, there is a need for careful decision making. The third issue is that of quality, that is ensuring that the service provided is what the patient requires. These needs informed the reorganisation. The forces, however, that drove the changes came from two simultaneous but different sources.

First the *Health of the Nation* directives (DoH 1991b, 1992), which were a delayed reaction to the Health for All strategy, succeeded in refocusing health care towards a health promotion and preventive service (Dept of Health 1992) (see Chapter 13). The other force emanated from those ideas contained in the government publication *Working for Patients*. This laid the foundation for the introduction of the internal market which later became enshrined in legislation through the 1990 NHS and Community Care Act. Second, *Working for Patients*, which was introduced throughout the 1980s with the intention of creating a managed market. By this

Activities

With your teacher or in a group discuss the following questions:

- How successful has the NHS has been in improving the health of the nation?
- Has the state assumed too much responsibility for the health and welfare of its citizens?
- What should be the responsibility of the individual?
- Is there too much administration within the current NHS?
- Is the NHS responsive to the needs of its consumers as in the private business sector?
- Is the NHS adequately resourced?

Having answered these questions discuss what further changes you feel could be made in the health service.

the government believed it would stimulate an incentive towards reducing even further the costs of health care through greater efficiency. To achieve this it was necessary for the government not to intervene excessively as the new markets emerged. At the same time, the government was obliged to retain responsibility for preventing a collapse of the markets that were stimulated. The difficulty therefore for government was achieving the correct balance.

REFERENCES

Able-Smith B 1994 An introduction to health policy, planning and financing. Longman, London

Advisory Committee for Management Efficiency in the National Health Service 1966 Management functions of hospital doctors. HMSO, London

Audit Commission 1992 Homeward bound: a new course for community health. HMSO, London

Baggott R 1994 Health and health care in Britain. St Martin's Press, Kent

Butler J 1993 Patients, policies and politics before and after Working for Patients. Open University Press, Buckingham

Central Health Services Council 1954 Report of the committee on the internal administration of hospitals. HMSO, London

Cmnd 7615 1979 Royal Commission on the National Health Service. HMSO, London

Davis B, Challis D 1986 Matching resources to needs in community care: an evaluated demonstration of a long-term care model. Gower, Aldershot

Dent M 1995 The new national health service: a case of postmodernism? Organisation Studies 16:875–899

Department of Health 1989a Working for patients. HMSO, London

Department of Health 1989b Caring for people: community care in the next decade and beyond. HMSO, London

Department of Health 1989c Health service management resource assumption and planning guidelines. Circular 89, HMSO, London

Department of Health 1991a The patient's charter. HMSO, London

Department of Health 1991b The health of the nation: a consultative document for health in England. (Cmnd 1523), HMSO, London

Department of Health 1992 The health of the nation: a strategy for health in England. (Cmnd 1986), HMSO, London

Department of Health and Social Security 1972a National health service reorganisation: England. (Cmnd 5055), HMSO, London

Department of Health and Social Security 1972b Management arrangement for the reorganised NHS. HMSO, London

Department of Health and Social Security 1979 Patients first. HMSO, London

Department of Health and Social Security 1983 NHS management inquiry. HMSO, London

Department of Health and Social Security 1984 Implementation of the NHS management inquiry report. Health Circular 84, HMSO, London

Department of Health and Social Security 1988 Review of resource allocation working party formula: final report of the NHS management board. HMSO, London

Gormley K 1996 Altruism: a framework for caring and providing care. International Journal of Nursing Studies 33(6):581–588

Griffith Sir R 1988 Community care: an agenda for action. HMSO, London

Guillebaud Committee 1956 The report of the committee of enquiry into the cost of the National Health Service. (Cmnd 9663), HMSO, London

Ham C 1985 Health policy in Britain. Studies in Social Policy. Macmillan Education, Basingstoke

Ham C 1991 The new National Health Service organisation and management. Radcliffe, Oxford

Hancock C 1995 Care in the year 2000. In: Jolly M, Brykczynska M Nursing beyond tradition and conflict. Mosby, London

Harrison S 1988 Managing the National Health Service: shifting the frontier. Chapman and Hall, London

James A 1994 Managing to care: public services and the market. Longman, London

Klein R 1989 The politics of the National Health Service, 2nd edn. Longman, London

Levitt R, Wall A, Appleby J 1995 The reorganised National Health Service. Chapman and Hall, London

Lister J 1988 Cutting the lifeline: the fight for the NHS. Journeyman, London

Medical Services Review Committee 1962 A review of the medical services in Great Britain. Social Assay, London

Ministry of Health 1962 A hospital plan for England and Wales. (Cmnd 1604), HMSO, London

Ministry of Health 1966 Report of the committee on senior nursing staff structure. HMSO, London

Owen D 1988 Our NHS. Pan, London

Ranade W 1994 A future for the NHS? Health care in the 1990s. Longman, London

Scottish Health Services Council 1966 Administrative practice of hospital boards in Scotland. HMSO, Edinburgh. Cited in: Harrison S 1988 Managing the National Health Service: shifting the frontier. Chapman and Hall, London

Sines D 1995 Organised care. In: Basford L, Slevin O 1995 Theory and practice of nursing: an integrated approach to health care. Campion Press, Edinburgh

WHO 1993 Evaluation of recent changes in the financing of health services. WHO, Geneva

The mixed economy of health care

8

Fred Sutton

At the end of this chapter the student will be able to:

- **describe the changes in government legislation**
- **understand what is meant by an internal market**
- **understand the different providers of health care**
- **discuss the different types of health care providers**

Introduction

Throughout the 1980s the Conservative government attempted to increase the effectiveness of the National Health Service and introduced a range of reforms. The aim of this chapter is to describe these reforms and those of the early 1990s. It will describe their net effect on the provision of health care and the introduction of other sectors outside of the public sector, as well as the expectations of the government concerning these sectors and the limitations on them.

Towards the end of the 1980s the government decided that the best way to achieve increased effectiveness in the NHS was through managerial reform and the establishment of an internal market. The series of managerial reforms that they introduced were intended to bring a more business minded attitude to the NHS, so that there would be more concern over efficiency and costs. This was followed by a set of structural reforms, leading to the establishment of internal markets, with the divorce of providers from purchasers. The internal market also achieves the earlier objectives, but along with this should increase choice for consumers of health care through competition other than on price. Increased choice is supposed to come about by competitive pressure similar to that found in commercial enterprises. In 1988 a community care proposal was put forward which stated that there should also be a move towards a mixed market of care providers, incorporating private and voluntary organisations. This was then extended to the entire NHS in the 1989 White Paper entitled *Working for Patients*.

THE MIXED MARKET

The 1989 White Paper *Working for Patients* reported the findings of the government's review of the NHS, and set out their proposals for the future. The government proposed to establish a mixed market for health service provision, including both the public and the private sectors. Market mechanisms would be introduced to the NHS in order to achieve their objectives, although the underlying principle of the NHS, that it would be funded through public taxation, would remain. This was the final stage of a process of reform which had begun with the introduction of general management in 1984, following the findings of the 1983 Griffith Report, which called for an NHS management board, and the move towards a more business management orientation. The Griffith Report also called for the introduction of performance indicators, in order to give a clear picture of the relationship between the budget allocated to clinical units and the work performed by their professional providers. This would lead to the publication of statistics on resource consumption and the service output, which in turn would highlight areas with potential problems (Saltman & Von Otter 1992).

One of the main aims of Thatcherism was the extension of the private market in all sectors of the economy (including the health care market), in the belief that the private sector would increase efficiency through competition. As part of this programme the existing nationalised industries were dismantled into smaller units and sold to the private sector in order to bring about an element of competition. The White Paper was perceived as a way of extending this ethos throughout the NHS by introducing an 'entrepreneurial spirit'. District authorities would continue to receive a public budget, but now they would no longer be the sole provider of services. The district authority would, however, also become a purchasing agent, and would seek out the 'best' care it required from various sources, whether public, private or voluntary. The best care would be in terms of quality as well as price, although the definition was somewhat vague: 'Health authorities carrying out their new role as purchasers rather than providers of care will buy in services from the private sector if it offers a better deal than is available from NHS hospitals' (DoH 1989, p. 68).

Activities

- In your school library review what is meant by the term mixed market and discuss your findings with your colleagues.
- List the areas in health and social care services that are provided by the private sector.

PRIVATISATION

Patients First (DHSS 1979) enabled the government to put pressure on regions to pursue privatisation policies. The key areas were clear. First the government wished to stimulate a greater role for the private sector in the area of community care for the elderly and people with mental health problems through private nursing homes and residential accommodation. Second it wished to stimulate the contracting of hotel services (such as laundry, catering and domestic work) out to private firms.

Traditionally the market for private health care was perceived by the public as a supplementary or complementary service to that which already existed in the statutory sector. It was marketed by companies as a service to those with the ability to pay as either a higher quality of care or a way of avoiding protracted waiting times for treatment. The private sector therefore became attractive to those who could afford to pay in spite of the obvious drawback of having to pay twice for services. However, even those who were well off realised that private schemes alone could not meet the costs of some chronic or even some acute conditions.

The image of the private sector gradually changed and became increasingly portrayed, during this period, as a service offering an equal and possibly more accessible service. The government argued that the private sector was just another strand of the whole package of available services, including those from the existing statutory and emerging voluntary sector. In taking this view the government was saved from the accusation that wealthier people had better access to health services than the poor, which would have been against the principle of equity. The mixed market policy was strengthened further by the government's argument that the income generated from the private sector allowed more resources to be channelled into the statutory sector.

Activities

- Discuss with your teacher the factors that made it necessary for the government to introduce privatisation policies into health and social care.
- Describe the net effects of this policy, remembering to support your arguments with statistical evidence.

Private residential care

The most significant growth in the government's privatisation policy was in the area of medium to long term care of elderly people and those with learning disabilities. By the turn of the 1980s the voluntary and private sector had overtaken the statutory provision for these two population groups. The origins of this policy can be traced

to a period of sharp economic decline in the mid-1970s which led to a reduction in the amount of money payable to local authorities in England and Wales and to health and social services boards in Northern Ireland. Regions could not meet the demand for services and, as a result, voluntary organisations took on a degree of responsibility for this area. To achieve this, they persuaded the government to allocate some additional money as supplementary benefits. This allowed individuals without sufficient means to purchase voluntary sector residential accommodation for themselves (Darton & Wright 1993).

Although it was voluntary organisations that led the campaign, the private sector quickly became the main beneficiaries in this new arrangement. While there was a rapid growth in this form of service it was at the expense of statutory provided residential homes and NHS long term hospital beds (Laing 1991). This later became known as the 'perverse incentive'. This arrangement caused considerable concern among elderly people and policy analysts because there was a fear that people were not placed in the setting most appropriate to their current or future needs. The report of the Audit Commission (1986) also criticised the perverse incentive and social services because the system encouraged elderly people to enter independent nursing homes rather than trying harder to maintain them in their own homes.

The use of residential or nursing home placements is considered to be inappropriate by those who advocate ordinary living as suitable for all. There was also criticism of the differential between income support for nursing home care and that for residential home care, which encouraged the placing of people who did not need nursing care into nursing homes rather than residential accommodation. The extent of misplacement was not addressed, and it still remains a difficult issue to resolve because of the great variety of reasons for which elderly people enter all types of residential accommodation (Darton & Wright 1993, Davis & Challis 1986). However, the system was eventually discontinued following the implementation of the National Health

Service and Community Care Act. Under the new arrangements, statutory support for a person entering nursing home care was only provided after a rigorous assessment and if it was demonstrably obvious that the individual required this form of service.

Activities

With your colleagues:

- Write brief notes on the term 'perverse incentive'.
- Discuss the reasons why the government used the perverse incentive as a means of stimulating a private sector in residential and nursing home services.

HOSPITAL SERVICES

Under the new Act hospitals would be allowed to opt out of the service and become self-governing institutions under the authority of a non-profit trust. The opted-out hospital would then be expected to sell its services to district health authorities in order to obtain patients. The hospital could also market itself at the privately insured. Self-governing hospitals could have direct contracts with their staff and also control their operating and capital decisions. The only constraints on hospitals entering into this type of arrangement were that they were required to have a system of medical audit and were obliged to continue to provide core services if no alternatives existed in the area. The third major change set out in the White Paper was that GPs were given control over part of their patients' annual acute care hospital budget. GPs, it was thought, would then send their patients to those hospitals providing the most cost-effective care, in order to maximise the amount of care they could purchase with their budgets.

COMMUNITY CARE

Community care services achieved a higher profile during the 1980s, partly because of the increased expenditure on social services due to increased demand for hospital and residential care services by the ageing population. Along with this was the Conservative government's drive towards care in the community and the reduction of long stay wards, particularly psychiatric wards. The belief behind this was that it would be more beneficial for people to be treated in a home setting as opposed to being institutionalised.

Community care has been defined by the Conservative government as the 'means of providing the services and support which people who are affected by problems of ageing, mental illness, or disability need to be able to live as independently as possible in their own home, or in "homely" settings in the community'.

In 1986 an Audit Commission report identified various problems which prevented the development of an effective community care service for dependent people. These included the organisational fragmentation between the various authorities such as health, social security, local authorities and voluntary groups; the lack of any bridging finance to move from an institutional to a community-based system; perverse payment incentives which actually encourage the use of residential care; and inadequate staffing arrangements. The commission felt that better value could be obtained from the existing arrangements.

Local authorities and community care

The White Paper, Caring for People, in 1989 moved that local authority social service departments should take the lead role in the provision of community care. The underlying philosophy

Box 8.1 Community care

The key components of community care should be:

- services that respond flexibly and sensitively to the needs of individuals and their carers
- services that allow a range of options for consumers
- services that intervene no more than is necessary to foster independence
- services that concentrate on those with greatest need

in the White Paper was to create services that were more sensitive to the needs of their users and carers, and which would give them more choice. This was an ideological shift to the provision of services from need, rather than providing services which people then have to fit into. The local authorities were not to provide the services themselves; services would be provided by a mixed economy, based largely on the private, voluntary and not-for-profit sectors. Local authorities were to become purchasers of care through the allocation of funds, and they would then have a declining role in direct service provision. Social services were to set out their strategy for achieving all this through a new system of community care plans. Local government also took over financial responsibility for those seeking support for people in residential homes, over and above their entitlement to general social security benefits. The introduction of the independent sector into the market for health care provision would establish a quasi market. The thought behind this was that state provision would be replaced by the more competitive independent services (Hoyes & Mean 1991).

These proposals were enacted through the NHS and Community Care Act of 1990, which was to be implemented in April 1991. The implementation of the Act was beset by problems, and was subsequently delayed, over the grounds that local authorities would not be ready in time. It was then decided that rather than introduce the policy in one go, it would be introduced over 3 years, to allow local authorities the time to implement the requirements.

Activity

With your colleagues discuss the benefits of community care policies for specific client groups.

The NHS and Community Care Act 1990

As we have seen, the idea behind community care was that it should be geared to the needs of the individual and carer; that social services should assess the community care needs of the locality and be organisers and purchasers of non-health care services, including residential and nursing homes. In practice, the Griffith Report (1988) found that social services departments and voluntary groups were having difficulty with funding problems at a local level. The report advocated that social services should be responsible for arranging care packages for individuals using a system of case management, where a person would be allocated a case-worker who would assess their care needs and tailor a care plan accordingly. The responsibility for medically required community health services would remain with the health authorities.

The NHS and Community Care Act 1990 emphasised the role of putting service users at the centre of those services, to be involved in the development of plans for reorganising community care services. This was partly as a result of acknowledging that resources are limited, and an infinite range of services could not be delivered. In this case, then a good quality basic service would be the best starting point. With this in mind the involvement of users in the planning and operation of services should help to achieve the best services that meet real user needs for the limited resources.

Private provision of community care

Consecutive Conservative governments tried to promote the private provision of community care in a number of ways. Voluntary organisations received an increase in funding from central government. Health authorities were urged to cooperate with them, and in 1985 voluntary organisations were included in the joint planning process. There was an indirect promotion of the informal sector by emphasising that the care of the elderly and other vulnerable groups was a community responsibility, as opposed to a state liability. Changes in the social security regulations in 1980 allowed the elderly to claim social security to cover the costs of residential care, which was also partly responsible for the explosion of private residential care (Baggot 1994).

Costs

Prior to the changes in community care, community care services for groups such as the elderly, those with learning difficulties and the mentally ill had tended to be institution based, and were funded either directly by the NHS or by local authorities (unfortunately they also tended to be underfunded). The implementation of care in the community was to remove these institutions and replace the care they offered with care in the community. People would then be moved out of long stay hospital beds, and reintegrated back into the community. People would have their needs assessed and a care plan formulated, so that they would be able to remain in their own homes.

The costs of long term care for the elderly, those with physical or learning disabilities and people with a mental illness have increased, despite the policy of transferring people from long stay hospitals to the community. The costs to the DSS of residential care for those unable to live independently have also escalated. Demographic trends indicate a continuing increase in the number of frail and very old people, many of whom live alone and are therefore likely to become more dependent on social and health services. This will have implications for the future costs of long term care. Although people may be able to live in their own homes for a longer period with the help of domiciliary services, they may well still end up in residential care at a later date (Smith 1993).

Activities

- Discuss the changes in community care legislation.
- Highlight potential problem areas for the future.

HEALTH CARE PROVISION

Health care provision is split into two areas, statutory and non-statutory health care. Statutory health care is that care which is provided mainly by the public sector, whereas non-statutory health care is provided by the independent sector. The public sector is that part of the social services which is financed and managed by the state. Traditionally, public services have tended to be established in areas where there were few (or no) alternatives, or they were formed to replace alternatives which were deemed unsatisfactory.

One of the arguments in favour of a public health sector is that, where there are minimum standards to maintain, requiring either a general regime or residual provision to plug the gaps, state provision best ensures that those standards are universal. Another argument for public services is that, where there are sensitive areas, such as the protection of children in social work, it is largely perceived that these services are best provided by a state body, which can be regulated and which is publicly accountable.

One of the problems with public sector health provision is that it has a tendency to be based in hospitals, where economies of scale can be accrued. This has led to care services being formulaic in nature with problems in establishing care services that are community based. Other sectors, such as the independent sector, may be better at providing some sorts of care, since they are potentially more flexible.

Activity

It has been argued that the public sector has always been a safety net that supports people during difficult times. Discuss with your colleagues whether this still applies following the implementation of community care policies.

Box 8.2 Mixed economy of care

- Statutory sector
- Private sector
- Voluntary sector

THE INDEPENDENT SECTOR

The independent sector covers a number of broad areas which, although they may have some similarities, can be quite different. It includes the private sector, the voluntary sector and the informal sector. Within each of these sectors there is a wide variety of different organisations, with different agendas and motivations. There has been a trend under the Thatcher/Major administrations to argue that the private sector is always the best method of distributing resources. Rather than providing people with the services per se, it is better to finance them with the opportunity to exercise choice over what they want. This then leads to a service that is consumer led, rather than led by the supplier. With a supplier led service so-called consumers have to fit themselves into whatever care is provided, even if it is not exactly what they require.

With a consumer led service, the sector will provide services that are genuinely required due to the nature of competition (that is, if they do not provide what is required, consumers will look elsewhere). The idea of a consumer led service ignores the tendency in the private market for organisations to congregate where there is greater need, leading to an over-supply in certain geographical areas, and an under-supply in others which are not so profitable because of low demand in those areas or the expense of delivering care to them. Along with geographical regions, there may be some types of care for which demand is low, which again will be ignored by the private sector.

The voluntary sector

The voluntary sector is composed of a number of organisations which range from small local societies to large very professional agencies and nationally known charities such as the NSPCC. Along with providing certain services, voluntary agencies can be instrumental in change due to pressure group activity. The kind of services and activities that they are involved in often depend on the size of the organisation. One of the main problems with the services provided by voluntary organisations is that services tend to be provided wherever the volunteers are based, as opposed to whether there is genuine need. This can lead to a wealth of volunteer groups in the more well-to-do liberal middle class areas, with a dearth of provision in the inner cities and in rural areas.

Informal care

The informal caring sector consists of the care that is provided informally by communities, friends and neighbours. This sector has increased in size and importance over recent years. The increase in private care provision and the discharge of people from institutions into the community has led to a greater emphasis on the role of carers. The experience of community care has shown the limitations of the other sectors in the provision of necessary care, with most of the care being provided by informal carers. The actions of the informal sector are not seen to cost the authorities any money, and so this would seem to be a very efficient way of organising care. However, although there may be no direct cost to society, there is an indirect cost, both through the loss of production and through increased strain on the carers (Spicker 1995).

Activities

- Carry out a literature review of the term informal care.
- Carry out a critique of an evidence based article on the subject of informal care and discuss the findings with your colleagues.

Non-statutory organisations

The independent sector includes all non-statutory organisations. It is made up of voluntary non-profit and private for-profit organisations. The organisations under these two rather broad umbrellas have different objectives.

These two broad areas can not be distinguished just by the fact that one is motivated by profit, whilst the other is not. This would give the impression that all one sector cares about is money, whereas the other does not care about money at all. This is not the case, as both sectors have to cover their costs and both have an interest in the quality of care they provide. In the private health care market there has been an increased attention towards the quality of care provided, whereas the voluntary sector has become more concerned over budgets and cost saving. So the belief that they are dichotomised has reduced, and rather than being polar opposites, they have come some way to sharing common factors.

Funding

The way the two sectors are funded and can attract funding are also different. Charities are dependent on voluntary contributions, although they are in a better position to attract subsidies, especially tax subsidies, than non-profit and for-profit organisations. The problem with being dependent on voluntary contributions is that there is no guarantee of how much will be collected for any given year. This can lead to difficulties in planning for the future and problems with attracting loans and capital injections. Along with this, the position of subsidies is not always concrete, and can be subject to change. As fund raising is a volatile affair, charities are subject to changes in the amount that they can collect, which will be dependent on factors outside their control such as recessions or the introduction of the national lottery. Some of the very large voluntary organisations and private operators will have their own well developed advice and support infrastructure. This will mean that they have a more secure basis and may also have the financial capacity to cover losses or entry costs over a number of years.

Private sector expansion

The private health care system has expanded greatly over the last 10–15 years. In 1979 only 4% of the population were covered by private health insurance; this had risen to 13% of the population by the 1990s. The Thatcher govern-

ment pursued policies which encouraged privatisation, and introduced moves to increase the size of the private health care market. In 1981 employers were allowed to set health insurance premiums against corporation tax and tax relief on private health insurance as a fringe benefit was introduced in the same year for employees earning less than £8500 a year. Along with this there was the reduction in NHS patients for dentists, the removal of free eye tests, increase in prescription charges, medicines being removed from the list of those approved by the NHS and therefore needing to be paid for in full. All these have helped to stimulate the private health care market.

As well as people having private health care insurance, many individuals pay directly for private health care without the benefit of insurance schemes. In 1986, just over a fifth of private patients, excluding abortions, were self-financing. Patients also pay directly for low cost treatments, such as over the counter medicines. Along with this there has also been a boom in purchasing care from the 'alternative' health sector.

Private health care and the NHS are not entirely divorced. Consultants have been allowed to practise private medicine since the NHS was set up. There are also private wards and beds in the NHS, and in fact the NHS has the largest share of private beds in the UK. So the relationship between the public and private health sector is not strictly dichotomous (Baggot 1994).

Activities

- Discuss the different providers of health care.
- Discuss the benefits of the different providers.
- Describe areas of care provision which would be best provided by each sector.
- Discuss areas which you think should remain solely in the public sector.

The contribution of charities and voluntary bodies to the NHS

Ever since the NHS was established there has

been charitable involvement, largely through the raising of funds (mainly aimed at medical research) and in the provision of supplementary services for patients. This involvement has increased over the past 20 years, and we are now at the position where charities and voluntary bodies no longer just provide optional extras, but also provide funds for core services, and through fund raising appeals contribute to hospital capital and running costs.

Residential care

The supply of residential care from the private sector has increased dramatically in recent times, especially in the provision of long term care of the elderly. Private provision is also significant in other areas of long term care, such as mental illness. Commercial and voluntary residential homes now supply well over half the places available in the UK. During the 1980s, the number of places available in local authorities increased slightly and those provided by charities fell, whereas those provided by the commercial sector more than quadrupled, although many of the private places are funded through the public sector.

Home care

One of the main aims of the NHS and Community Care Act 1990 was to remove the incentives towards residential care and stimulate the use of home care. This could be seen in one of two ways. It could be argued that to increase the use of home care would fulfil the criteria of increasing care in the community, enabling people to remain in their own homes for as long as possible. Or stimulating home care could be regarded as more of a cost-cutting device, as it saves the costs of residential care and relies on provision of care by the informal sector. The choice of home care presupposes that there is an organisation supplying home care in that location, from whom the purchasing authorities may purchase this care.

The nature of domiciliary care raises the problem of whether purchasers have all the necessary information to purchase the best care that is around, assuming that quality is taken into the equation. Much domiciliary care takes place behind closed doors, in individual units, mostly in people's own homes, so it is difficult to gauge the quality and the nature of the care from the outside. Normally it is consumers who go to the providers for a product, with domiciliary care the providers go to the consumers. This fact alone means that the providing of domiciliary care can be very time-consuming, which may be a disincentive for volunteers to get involved.

The progress towards the development of a market in domiciliary care has been slow, for several different reasons. There is a feeling that social care is different to other modes of care, and there is the existence of other priorities and incentives. Local authorities would prefer there to be a greater supply of domiciliary care from the voluntary sector, but the very nature of domiciliary care may act against this. There may well be a large supply of care that is provided by families, which is not recognised. The majority of private domiciliary care is supplied on an individual basis. If there is a change in the market of domiciliary care two questions arise. Will there be a shift from family provided care to that from the independent sector if the quality is improved and the value for money is increased? If there is a change in the market will this lead to an increase in the provision of actual care or will it result in a substitution from one sector to another?

ASSISTING INDEPENDENT LIVING

One of the main thrusts behind the NHS and Community Care Act was to help people live as independently as possible, either in their own homes or in residential or nursing homes. People will have their needs assessed and planned as a care package. Responsibility for planning this care will fall mainly on local authority social services departments, who will work closely with health authorities to ensure that there are joint planning and service arrangements at every level.

Community care

Whilst care in the community rather than in long stay hospitals has been central to government policy, the emptying of long stay hospitals has not been matched by equal provision in the community. Homelessness among discharged mental patients and other vulnerable people has increased. The resources that have been saved by the emptying of long stay beds has stayed within the NHS, and has not gone towards the establishment of community care services. One of the main objections to the policy has been that without proper resources the policy implementation would have a watered down effect. Due to the nature of the funding from different budgets, money from the savings to the NHS should have been moved into local services in order for the policy to be effective and achieve its aims.

Residential care

The changes in social security rules and limits on local authority spending have led to an increase in private residential care. Between 1979 and 1991 the amount spent by social security to meet residential or nursing home fees rose dramatically from £10 million to £1.8 billion. There has been an increase in private care homes along the south coast, with a shortage in inner city areas. This is partly due to the decline of the traditional British holiday market, and the moving of traditional bed and breakfast hotels to some form of residential care.

Some who could have stayed at home with a little domiciliary support have been effectively institutionalised. Health and social services authorities have turned to independent sector homes, as these will be funded from the social security budget. The NHS has shed over 8000 continuing care beds over the past 10–15 years, as those no longer requiring acute hospital care have been transferred to nursing homes. Now those who need residential care will have to be assessed by their social services department. The assessment is intended to ensure that the individual's needs are fully considered and that

the appropriate care arrangements are made. The full cost of that care will be met by the local authority, whoever actually provides it. Where community health and nursing services are needed in addition to care provided within the home, the health service will pay.

Cooperation between social services and health authorities

The changes have obliged social service departments and health authorities to work together to ensure that there are agreements on assessments, hospital discharge procedures and a range of other issues, including how GPs and primary health care teams fit in. In each social services authority area, agreements must be reached with all the local health authorities.

In 1992 Virginia Bottomley announced the community care grant for the next three years, and at the same time also announced that the grants would only be available if councils had reached agreement before the end of the year on who would be responsible for placing people in nursing homes, and on the integration of hospital discharge arrangements with assessment procedures. The government tried to stimulate the independent sector by announcing that two thirds of the community care grant must be spent on the independent sector. The government also expected the independent sector to expand into domiciliary care, although the requirements for councils to register and inspect privately run homes were not extended to domiciliary care.

The drive towards mixed provision of care by local authorities and the independent sector

Activities

- Discuss with your friends how government policy encourages frail older people to remain at home as long as possible, rather than unnecessarily entering some form of residential care.
- Organise a seminar to discuss the net effects of community care policies on families of dependent older people.

means that local authorities have been going through the process, already experienced in the health services, of separating their purchasing and provider roles. Local authorities will still be direct providers where they have their own residential homes but increasingly they will be purchasing community care from the independent sector.

CHANGES IN FUNDING

Prior to 1993 there were four main sources of help and funding for people for health services. Health authorities were able to offer district nursing and other community health services, while local authorities could offer personal care assistance at home and arrange for a variety of other help, such as housing adaptations which would be paid for by their disabled facilities grants. The DSS provided disability benefits as well as other social security benefits. People could apply to the Independent Living Fund, if they had severe disabilities, if they needed to purchase extra care.

Previously, nursing and residential care were funded through social security money, which was available to individuals through means tested benefits. This money was now paid in a lump sum to local social services departments, by means of a formula which determines how much money they should need, which means that there is now a limit to the amount of money available to pay for residential care.

Local authority spending on social services for home care is ultimately governed by the government-set standard spending assessment (SSA) and money raised through the community charge. The SSA is a complex series of calculations that uses social indicators to determine the likely amount of social services needed in a county or borough. Many authorities now make a charge for domiciliary care services through some form of means test.

The DSS has a range of means tested benefits: IS, housing and community charge benefit, family credit and so on, plus non means tested benefits such as attendance and mobility allowance (now largely incorporated into disabled living allowance), invalidity benefit, severe disablement allowance and the carers' benefit and invalid care allowance.

For those getting attendance allowance or the higher care component of the disabled living allowance, and requiring extra care assistance, the Independent Living Fund (ILF) could offer payments up to £400 a week in some cases. However, in November 1992 the fund was closed to new applicants, although it continued to pay existing recipients. Its successor body can be approached only if the local authority is already providing services to the value of the average local residential fee. However, unlike the ILF, the new fund is not open to new applicants over retirement age (George 1993).

From April 1993 more people were to be assessed for unmet needs and to be provided with domiciliary services. Without the automatic payments of DSS money for residential care, more people are expected to stay in the community, mainly at home. These people will now require domiciliary services.

The transfer of community care funds to local authorities requires them to have joint assessment and care planning arrangements with local health bodies, usually the district health authority, but also other purchasers like GP fundholders.

The local authorities have the ultimate responsibility for assessing the care needs of people and for carrying out a test of their resources. Clients should have a coordinated service from community nursing, personal care assistants and so on. Local authorities will still be able to charge clients for any non-health services that they provide. Under the terms of the transfer of community care money, local authorities are expected to purchase the majority of home care services, rather than providing them themselves.

THE HEALTH CARE MARKET

The 1990 NHS and Community Care Act established the framework for a market in health care, funded and managed by the state. Within this market purchasing agencies contract health care from provider organisations, on behalf of their clients (i.e. the population). Although the policy was initially described as establishing an internal market in the public NHS, later government statements have made it plain that it very much encourages trading across NHS and private sector boundaries. Within this mixture of public and private provisions, health authorities may find it more economical, for example, to purchase a greater part of their continuing care for the elderly from private nursing homes. Some GPs are already referring the majority of their patients to private hospitals, and private insurance companies are taking advantage of the improved pay bed facilities offered by NHS trusts.

Along with the NHS using private services, there has been a movement the other way, with private capital being used in the NHS. This raises new accountability issues not normally encountered in the health service's trading relationship with the private sector. The use of private capital generates risks which can neither be easily calculated nor easily regulated. Along with this, in some cases it may be more expensive to use private capital as opposed to using public capital. The extent of the commitment of NHS resources is to an extent unknown. It may be possible for the state to regulate the internal market of the NHS, but how can it regulate the relationship between that public market and the private financial market? The NHS will still have to demonstrate value for money, but where the private sector is in the lead it will no longer be necessary to consider a theoretical alternative funded wholly by the NHS.

The preoccupation of the government is how best to ensure that public money and the public interest are adequately protected through the use of appropriate systems of accountability (Salter 1995).

Social service provision

Social service provision is supposedly a local government matter. Although local government decides how much will be spent each year on their social services, they are constrained by their budgets, set by central government, which allow little room for manoeuvre. Central government makes the decisions determining how much money will be available for the personal social services; these central decisions are made with only a broad and technical reference to social need. Central government also decides the duties and objectives of the services; local authorities must then do the best they can to fulfil their legal obligations within the funds available to them. In effect, the only way they can improve a service by spending more on it is by cutting other services.

Social need

Publicly funded personal social services exist to help the most frail and vulnerable in our society. Both the NHS and Community Care Act 1990 and the Children Act 1989 require local authorities to monitor and to meet 'need'. The Children Act requires authorities to 'take reasonable steps' to identify the extent to which there are children in need within their area, and specifies areas of relevant need. The community care legislation goes further, asking authorities to produce annual figures of the number in their communities likely to require services and to submit plans to the secretary of state indicating how they propose to meet the need.

There are few reasons why the supply of services should respond directly to changes in social need. Health education and social security services have both grown or shrunk in relation to need, but such a question is less meaningful when asked of personal social services. Local authority services have rarely been sufficient to offer assistance to more than a minority of those likely to be defined as in need of help. It is argued that the state should only provide a proportion of the care demanded, and so there should not be a direct link between the demand and supply of public services.

It is well established that the vast amount of care work not done by the state is provided by families and through informal local communities. The notion of the family as a caring unit is in flux and under threat. Politicians have realised that small reductions in the supply of family care could have substantial costs for the public sector if it had to fill the gap.

Activities

- The government has said that money for care should follow patients. Discuss with your teacher what this means.
- List five examples in health care provision where this has had a major impact.

PROBLEMS FACING A MIXED MARKET

Domiciliary care

When purchasers are looking at the independent sector for the provision of domiciliary care they are met with a series of problems. They need to have an existing supply of care, from different sources, so that they can choose quality care at a reasonable price. For purchasers to make decisions between different services they need information about the services. They also need some way of evaluating the care provided, and need to know that the supply will be reliable. Without a number of different suppliers competing for contracts there will be no mechanism for ensuring low cost quality care. If there is just one supplier then there is a potential for a monopoly situation, where the cost and quality are decided by other means.

Private firms may be reluctant to enter the market for domiciliary care because they question the stability of the reforms. They may think that the reforms are political in nature and the internal market could be removed by a change of government. If the costs of entering the market are high, then they may be reluctant to start up if there is no guarantee that the situation will last long enough for them to recoup the initial setting up costs.

They may also have doubts concerning the finances that are available to local authorities. Considering that local authorities operate under a system of limited resources, there is no guarantee that the original spending plans on care will remain stable over the years. When savings are needed certain plans may be restricted to enable the resources to be spent elsewhere.

One of the areas that may be liable to cost cutting is the supply of domiciliary care to certain groups, by tightening up the eligibility criteria, thereby further destabilising projected market demand.

These reasons may lead to existing care providers, or potential care providers, waiting to see what will happen before they consider either expanding their services or entering into the market. Voluntary organisations may have other obstacles to entering the market. They may lack sufficient resources to develop the necessary paper work for bidding for contracts, or they may fear losing their independence by becoming liable to regulations imposed by the local authority. One of the potential problems with this is whether encouraging the voluntary sector to provide care will actually augment the stock of health care. It is possible that rather than providing extra services or increasing the overall supply, voluntary organisations will replace the care provided by local authorities.

Conclusion

For the NHS and Community Care Act to be effective, there has to be a large supply of services for people who live at home in order for there to be a competitive market. The competition between the different organisations in the independent sector should then provide quality services at low costs. This competitive spirit should lead to the supply of services being tailored to the needs of the service users, to encourage the local authorities to purchase their care services. At the present time this has not occurred; whether it will or not in the future is open to debate. It is possible that the 1980s increase in residential care may well be mirrored. However, this view is possibly over-optimistic, since the majority of the increase in residential care was from the private for-profit sector rather than from the whole of the independent sector, and at the time residential care was funded through the benefits system. If the supply of care is not there, despite the demand, then the supply of care has to be stimulated in some way. The regime of short term contracts for care will not help this situation, since short term contracts will not encourage organisations to take the necessary risks of setting up agencies to provide care.

The NHS and Community Care Act is based on the ideas of private commercial markets and management, yet the management of service provision is difficult, and many of the underlying assumptions about how markets operate in practice are redundant in this area. The idea of increasing competition to reduce costs may not work, and in fact may lead to increased costs. If providers of care are tendering for a large number of small contracts, then the work that goes into that tendering process may well lead to an increase in total costs, especially if not all the bids are successful, as the cost of tendering for the unsuccessful bids have to be covered in the successful ones.

Promotion of the independent sector is supposed to achieve greater efficiency and effectiveness in resource allocation. This should lead to improvements in value for money. The fact that there would be negotiations for care services would be expected to result in cheaper services, through the effects of competition. This has not necessarily taken place. What has been more

common is collaboration between a single purchaser and provider, as opposed to competition. With an imperfect market such as this it is more difficult for a local authority to achieve the most cost-effective care.

Promoting consumer choice cannot be achieved without encouraging the independent sector. Not only do they have to enter the market, but they also have to provide a range of care. A large independent sector does not necessarily lead to an increase in choice for consumers if the services provided are the same as those provided by the existing health authorities. If one of the goals of the Act is to achieve an increase in consumer choice, then this has to be included in the process of stimulating the supply side of health care services.

Activities

- Discuss the obstacles facing different providers of care who wish to enter the market.
- Discuss how they could be encouraged to enter into the market.

REFERENCES

Audit Commission 1986 Making a reality of community care. HMSO, London

Baggot R 1994 Health and health care in Britain. Macmillan, Basingstoke

Darton R, Wright K 1993 Changes in the provision of long-stay care, 1970–1990. Health and Social Care in the Community 1(1):11–25

Davis B, Challis D 1986 Matching resources to needs in community care: an evaluated demonstration of a long-term care model. Gower, Aldershot

Department of Health and Social Security 1979 Patients First. HMSO, London

Department of Health 1989 Working for patients. HMSO, London

Department of Health 1990 Caring for people. White Paper. HMSO, London

Department of Health 1990 Caring for people. Community

care in the next decade and beyond. Policy Guidance. HMSO, London

George M 1993 Community care act. Funding the Act. Nursing Times 89(5):24–25

Griffith, Sir R 1988 Community care: an agenda for action. HMSO, London

Hoyes L, Mean R 1991 Implementing the White Paper on community care: SAUS Publications

Laing W 1991 Empowering the elderly: direct consumer funding of care services. Institute of Economic Affairs, Health and Welfare Unit, London

Salter B 1995 The private sector and the NHS: redefining the welfare state. Policy and Politics 23(1):17–30

Saltman R B, Von Otter C 1992 Planned markets and public competition. Open University Press

Spicker P 1995 Social policy themes and approaches. Prentice Hall/Harvester Wheatsheaf

9 Disability

Kevin Gormley

At the end of this chapter the student will be able to:

- **define the term disability**
- **describe the changes in legislation for disabled people**
- **describe the changing focus of government policy for disabled people**
- **discuss the influence of government in meeting the changing needs of disabled people**
- **contrast the changing role of public services for disabled people**

Introduction

This chapter will assess the current government response towards meeting the needs of people with a disability.

Professional definitions of disability vary and generally reflect the diversity of interest in this particular policy area. Psychologists and educationalists consider disability in terms of intelligence testing, while health care workers such as nurses, physiotherapists or occupational therapists associate disability with environmental and physical barriers to performing daily living skills. Oliver (1996) provides a definition of disability that contains three elements:

- the presence of an impairment
- the experience of environmentally imposed restrictions
- self-identification as a disabled person.

Disability as an issue of social policy is concerned with all that disables, injures or physically handicaps. This definition in reality provides only a minimal interpretation of the real extent of disability. A disability can range from mild to severe and can be emotional, physical or intellectual. The person with a disability can be a child born with cerebral palsy, a teenager paralysed following a road traffic accident, a mother suffering the severest effects of rheumatoid arthritis or an older person with Alzheimer's disease.

Interest in disability issues began with the medical professions in the 18th century and gradually philanthropist reformers of the 19th century became more prominent. In the 1970s the disability rights movement, led by disabled people, transformed the traditional perception of the disabled community. They pressured for a change in the focus of services for disabled people and demanded equal access to all aspects of society as a fundamental civil right. The net effect of the movement has been a set of public policies known as disability care policy (Davidhizar 1997) (see Box 9.1).

The general public was surprised when, during the 1970s and 1980s, it became clear that there were militant persons with disabilities demanding equality of rights as citizens. Before this the general public assumed that disabled people were either incapable of organised concerted political action or else were content with their lot in terms of welfare and voluntary support. It appeared that if an individual had a problem, then society assumed that professionals (doctors, nurses, social workers) would satisfy her needs. Disability groups wished to highlight the fact

that they did not want this form of service to be the only option (Oliver 1996).

DISABILITY/IMPAIRMENT/HANDICAP

The word impairment focuses on a precise area of the body that is not fully functioning; disability reflects the individual reaction to the impairment, and the term handicap concentrates on the societal attitude and reaction to impairment. Therefore the main determinant as to whether or not a person is disabled is the way the individual interacts with her environment. The *International Classification of Impairment, Disabilities and Handicaps* of the World Health Organization (WHO 1980) makes the difference between these three concepts even more clear, though frequently all three terms are used interchangeably (see Box 9.2).

In spite of these clear guidelines, the term handicap has fallen into disrepute, particularly among the disabled population, principally because it is often used inappropriately. Frequently societies impose the term handicap on people with a disability regardless of whether or not they feel handicapped by the society in which they live (Batavia 1993).

Disability includes all the things that attempt to exclude people from society. These can range from prejudice to institutional discrimination. It is possible to appreciate that many of the

---

Box 9.1 Disability care policy

To understand this policy and how it differs from other policies, four points need to be considered:

- the dominant definition of disability
- the association of disability with health and able-bodied people
- the people who fit into this definition
- the more important disability policies that have been legislated, such as the Disability Discrimination Act

---

Box 9.2 The international classification of impairment, disabilities and handicaps of the World Health Organization (WHO 1980)

Disability: A person with a disability has a functional limitation that may be intellectual or physical. This limitation can result in a lack of ability to perform an activity in the manner or within the range considered normal for most people

Impairment: A person with a loss or abnormality of psychological, physiological or anatomical structure

Handicap: A person who encounters any form of disadvantage that is a direct result of an impairment or disability and limits the fulfilment of the person's normal role. A handicap is considered outside of other social factors which affect the role of individuals including age, gender, employment and cultural factors

social consequences that affect disabled people are not random but a rigid and systematic way of marginalising them. The Union of the Physically Impaired Against Segregation (UPIAS) agree that it is society that disables physically impaired people. In their view disability is something additional to impairment and they consider that disabled people are unnecessarily isolated and excluded from full participation within society. As a result, disabled people form a significant but oppressed minority group within society (UPIAS 1976).

Activities

- Discuss with your colleagues the difference between an impairment and a handicap.
- Make a list of the various forms of disabilities that you have encountered in your clinical practice.

Social and economic effects

People with a disability are not a homogenous group, their strengths and weaknesses differ widely and individual needs vary in complexity and require different kinds of help. In spite of these differences, all disabled people will have an interruption in their pattern and quality of life; if the disability becomes permanent it will cause additional disturbances in relationships and activities. Furthermore a person classified as disabled faces common social problems of stigma, marginalisation and discrimination in many areas of their daily living (Blaxter 1980, Hahn 1993, Szymanski & Trueba 1994).

Social effects

The term 'stigma' was used by the Ancient Greeks. At that time a stigma was usually a bodily sign that exposed something unusual or different about the moral status of a person. The stigmatised person usually had words or symbols burnt onto their body indicating clearly to the remainder of society that the person was, for example, a slave, a criminal, or suffering from a contagious disease. In modern society, although there is no requirement for a mark on the person's body, the categorisation of individuals continues. Usually through the treatment handed out to an individual, she is perfectly aware of her social identity or position in society. There is a belief within society that people with a disability who suffer the ignominy of a stigma are less than a whole person. A stigma remains something that is deeply discrediting and usually incurs exclusion from mainstream society and many forms of discrimination (Goffman 1984, p. 13).

Case 9.1

Most people have either witnessed or been directly exposed to some form of discrimination associated with disability. I remember a girl at the school that I attended who had lost a leg following a road traffic accident. At an inter-school swimming gala she won the butterfly event. However, following an investigation she was disqualified from the event. The reason for this, according to the judges, was because she had not kept two legs together. This was in some way supposed to have unfairly advantaged her over the remainder of the competitors.

Activities

- Describe what is meant by the term 'stigma'.
- From your life experience discuss with your colleagues a situation when you felt a person with a disability was made to feel uncomfortable.

There is evidence that at all stages of life the risk of chronic disability is consistently greater among the lower occupational groups. Alongside this there is evidence to suggest that disabled people are less able to access appropriate care and support (Titmuss 1963, Townsend & Davidson 1982). As the individual with a disability attempts to re-establish a normal lifestyle there is a residual effect on the life of a family.

While the disabled person's new lifestyle may suit the needs of the family, the wider society may perceive it as abnormal. Thus, in certain cases, an entire household unit can become disabled and socially isolated. For example, if a disabled person is unable to negotiate stairs in a household, sleeping and WC arrangements may require the conversion of a downstairs room. The presence of a commode in what was once a daytime living area can be embarrassing to people.

Economic effects

The economic implications of disability closely relate to a person's social circumstances. There is evidence of a correlation between disability and relative poverty. This relates to the additional costs incurred from the disability coupled with the loss of income. In the longer term, financial reserves become exhausted and any financial contributions from friends and family or past employers dwindle or cease. People with a disability frequently need more fuel, clothing, laundry, special equipment, diets, transport costs and paid support at home. Additionally, another member of the family often has to give up work to support the disabled family member (Smith 1996).

Structural changes in the labour market have had long term effects on employment opportunities for everybody, but they have had a particular impact on people with a disability. An examination of current earning levels shows a fall in demand for workers with a limited education and job skills. The reason for this is mainly because the manufacturing industrial base of the United Kingdom has been replaced by a 'high tech' service sector job market. This has increased the demand for well educated workers. The change has also had a mixed effect for disabled people. Given the fall in the demand for manual work, the presence of a physical disability is not as important as it once was, and thus highly skilled disabled people are finding greater employment opportunities. Conversely, it has limited the openings for other disabled people, especially those with either a mental health problem or learning difficulties, because

previously this group of people could have probably coped at some level in the traditional heavy industrial setting.

Disability Living and Working Allowance

The United Kingdom, along with the rest of Wester Europe, has in recent times had to face the problem of large numbers of people becoming unemployed. The social welfare response can be categorised into three groups:

- work-based interventions which provide opportunities for further training and branching out into a new career
- unemployment benefit which provides an income for those in between jobs
- disability benefit that provides a secure income for those so limited through their disability that they are unable to work.

The structures for Disability Working Allowances are described in the Disability Living Allowance and Disability Working Allowance Act 1991. Disability Living Allowance is the main source of income for people who have either a physical or psychological disability. To receive this allowance the disabled person must need attention or supervision from someone in order to meet their daily needs. It is a tax free benefit and is additional to other benefits that the disabled person may receive. Disability Allowance consists of two components: one for care needs and one for mobility and individual needs. This benefit replaced Mobility Allowance and Attendance Allowance (for those aged under 65 years) in April 1992.

There are a number of physical needs that entitle a person to the care component of the Disability Living Allowance. Lord Denning, in the Court of Appeal, gave a list of bodily functions that includes difficulty with: breathing, hearing, eating, walking, sitting, sleeping and eliminating (Box 9.3). The list does not include cooking, shopping or any of the other things that a member of the household generally does for the rest of the family. There are two key factors about the payment of Disability Allowance. First,

Box 9.3 Disability Living Allowance

Disability Living Allowance is allocated to people with the following bodily problems:

Breathing
Eating
Hearing
Walking
Sleeping
Eliminating

disabled people receive payments for potential risk as well as an actual risk of injury. For example in the case of people who have epilepsy, much of the supportive care is potential in that they need assistance only when a convulsion occurs. Second, assessment focuses on the needs of the claimant irrespective of whether supervision already occurs. Thus someone who is not supervised but needs to be would receive benefit whereas someone who is supervised, but does not need to be, would not qualify. Disabled people receive Disability Working Allowance if they are in low paid work. This allowance permits disabled people to participate in work and remain part of the community and avoid the isolating effects of their disablement. At the same time they avoid being penalised financially.

Activities

- Outline how the government attempts to meet the financial needs of a person with a disability.
- Contact a local support group for disabled people and find out whether they feel that this form of support is sufficient or appropriate.

MEDICAL MODEL OF DISABILITY

Most models that address the needs of disabled people associate the nature and extent of their problems with the limitations that exist as a residual consequence of disability. The models focus on how they are to lead a life with a physical, sensory or intellectual impairment. The medical and social care professions have

been particularly prominent in developing this idea. The medical model has led society to consider disability simply within the confines of the disease process, physical abnormality or personal trauma. This model has sometimes been referred to as the 'personal tragedy model' because, almost invariably, society's involvement has been only to express concern and sympathy to the disabled person and her family (French 1994). Within this framework two things happened. First, society was absolved from any responsibility to assist or support the disabled person. It appeared that the association of inequality and incapacity with disability was a roundabout way of blaming the disabled person for the discriminative practices rather than the rest of society. Second, this strategy failed to provide a valuable framework wherein disabled people could try to pick up the pieces and resume their life (Hales 1996).

Studies into the area of disability utilise a political strategy that encourages the debate to avoid the traditional personal tragedy model of physical impairment and limitation. Instead the political strategy promotes a consideration of the economic needs of disabled people as any other minority group, for example in being able to access training, education, employment and housing. The minority group argument suggests that persistent inequalities in society relate to social attitudes and negative public policies which, according to disabled groups, are the principal causes of problems for disabled people. It also attempts to reduce the social effects of disability, including the way disabled people interact with the able-bodied population and the negative attitudes that continue to persist (Hahn 1993). This revised political strategy has removed the functional limitation argument with some degree of success. Society now accepts that disabled people are the same as any other minority group who have to face prejudice and discrimination.

HEALTH OR SOCIAL CARE FOR DISABLED PEOPLE

Within the medical model a boundary exists that

separates services that are provided by either social care or health care services. It is an area of professional and policy tension, particularly in the area of caring for people with disabilities. The boundary is not a single element but a series of overlapping differences. These include areas such as payment for care, the nature of care and responsibility between various professional groups. Health care tends to have a high social status because of its link with the medical profession and high tech interventions that promote curing. In contrast, social care has a low status because it appears to be an area from which medicine has, to a certain extent, withdrawn. Social care is considered 'low tech' and includes people with a disability for whom there is little prospect of significant improvement in terms of a cure. In a survey carried out by Thorne (1993) on people with chronic disabilities, she describes how hospital staff gradually distanced themselves from patients. The staff used a range of strategies as a mechanism for withdrawing any long term responsibility for them. These include extended appointment dates, displaying a reduced optimism for progress and referral to support social care services (Thorne 1993, Twigg 1997).

Although the person with a disability may initially feel rejected, in the longer term it can be a positive move. It also reflects the wishes of disability groups. They contend that within the social care parameters new relationships can be formed with a focus on empowerment and independence. For a long time disabled groups have expressed concern about the over-medicalisation of what are essentially life problems. This view is supported by critics of excessive health care interventions, who suggest that when this occurs individuals tend to transfer onto health care staff the responsibility for many of society's intransigent problems (such as loneliness, family disharmony or isolation).

Fox (1990) argues that, as a result of technological progress, people living in Western societies unnecessarily defer health care issues to health care professionals. The criticism is not of the technology but its effect on our view of health as something that we depend on experts

and machines to provide for us. Illich (1976), a constant critic of the medicalisation of social problems, argues that social problems are very sensitive for the individual concerned. When this sensitivity combines with the high value that society places on health care it creates an unnecessary demand for health care – a demand that in the public mind only health care staff can solve. Illich describes this as a form of imperialism which is very difficult to oppose. According to Illich, this has perpetuated the mystique of health care and further reduces the potential for society to take responsibility for meeting the needs of people with disabilities.

Activity

Make brief notes on why groups of disabled people were unhappy with the medical model as a strategy for meeting their needs.

THE SOCIAL MODEL OF DISABILITY

In recent years disability lobbies have tried to undermine the dominant medical model and its definition of disability and the provision of care within that philosophy (Morris 1993, Oliver 1996). Out of this discontent a new social model has evolved that rejects the singular focus and responsibility of disability on the affected individual. It does not attempt to deny the existence of disability but relocates it within and as a part of society (Oliver 1996). Within the social model it is not individual limitation that is the problem but society's failure to adapt and move towards providing services that adequately meet the needs of disabled people.

The social model attempts to disentangle the disempowering elements of the medical model of disability and replace it with a social or collective responsibility strategy. It has two objectives. First, it wishes to reduce the negative features traditionally associated with being disabled. As a replacement it supports new ideas of inclusiveness and integration, where disabled people

Table 9.1 Models of disability (adapted from Oliver (1996))	
Individual model	**Social model**
Personal responsibility	Society involvement
Medical control	Personal empowerment
Prejudice	Discrimination
Control	Choice
Care	Rights
Individual adaptation	Social change
Personal tragedy theory	Social discrimination

avoid marginalisation and are made to feel a part of society. Second, the model would like to adjust the negative attitudes of society so that, on the one hand, disabled people will be able to enjoy equal rights and privileges, and, on the other hand, accept their responsibilities to contribute and play their role as good citizens (Pfeiffer 1993) (Table 9.1).

Activities

- Discuss with a group of your colleagues why it is important that society adapts in order to meet the needs of people with a disability.
- List any five areas where you feel society continues to marginalise people with a disability.

DISABILITY ORGANISATIONS

There are two distinct types of disability organisation, both of which evolved around the end of the 19th century. These are organisations of disabled people and organisations for disabled people. The control and management of organisations of disabled people is firmly in the hands of disabled people, whereas able-bodied people manage organisations for disabled people. The original organisations of disabled people in the United Kingdom were the British Deaf Association (founded in 1890) and the National League for the Blind (founded in 1898). Organisations for disabled people tended to hold the same political ideals as their sister organisations but were more influential in attracting financial and political support. They usually arose following a disaster or period of political turmoil. The Royal British Legion was a good example. It was set up to meet the needs of those injured and left with long term disabilities following the two great wars. Another similar support group appeared in the early 1960s to help those affected by the drug Thalidomide, prescribed by doctors for women during pregnancy as an antiemetic. As everybody knows, the drug caused catastrophic physical damage to unborn babies. These two groups have been particularly significant in the 20th century in demanding equal and civil rights for people with specifically defined disabilities (Barnes 1992, French 1994, Scott-Parker 1989).

There is similarity in the goals of the disability movement and other minority rights groups. Disabled people are striving to find a social order of equality that engages ideas of acceptance and tolerance. At the same time, underlying the debate, all minority groups accept that they are different and therefore need different treatment (for example women require crèche facilities, disabled people require structural changes to buildings). The paradox lies in the fact that disabled people require both equality and difference. They need equal treatment most of the time but in special circumstances, where they are genuinely different, they need special provision (Davis 1996, Watson 1993).

HEALTH WITHIN DISABILITY

Throughout life mankind pursues a healthy and meaningful existence and, for the most part, ill-health or disability is only a passing thought or small dimension of life's experiences. Disability is characterised by the term incapacity and its threat to self-care (Tannahill 1990). It is because health is linked to positive aspects of life and its obvious joys that disability conjures pictures of sadness, isolation and despair. Redman (1993) suggests that the nature of health needs to be reviewed and considered from a broader perspective and that existing parameters are narrow and unsuitable to modern health care systems. Recognising this dilemma for disabled people, Orem (1991) uses the term 'inner well-ness' to describe feelings of self-worth, contentment and fulfilment of one's ideal that a person may have in spite of the presence of a disability. According to Orem, when one considers ill-health or disability as a part or component of health it can lead to the expansion of human potential and facilitate personal growth and development specifically through increased self-awareness.

In the past, nurses and other health care professionals tended to ignore the lived experience of disability from the perspective of the individual. Health care services have traditionally preferred to focus on problem identification and the alleviation of signs and symptoms that present as a result of the disability. Moch (1989) suggests that this attitude has encouraged a perspective of health as being the inverse of ill-health. In her health promotion model Nola Pender (1990) rejects the notion of a health/ill-health continuum. Such a view of health detracts from the potential of people with disabilities to achieve high levels of health in their terms. According to Pender, ill-health is another human experience from which individuals can modify and adapt their lifestyle (Pender 1990).

Parse (1990) suggests that health is a process of unfolding experiences where each individual creates their own limits of health which are constantly changing throughout their life experience. Parse provides a realigned interpretation of health. She suggests that its existence may or may not be present but either way the presence of disease or disability is not a determinant. Parse rather philosophically goes on to describe health as a personal commitment wherein only I know me and my own living values. Therefore I constitute my own health with my mutual interconnections with the world.

Studies have found that people with disabilities have equal or higher levels of life satisfaction than people without any disability. This view confirms the results of an investigation of people with spinal cord injuries and other forms of disability (Rodgers & Marini 1994, Theuerkauf & Carpenter 1992). These studies highlight the capability of people with disabilities to quickly

learn to make adaptations to their lives. As a result, people with disabilities soon gain control of their own environment and are able to take charge of their destinies.

Stuifbergen and colleagues (1990) interviewed people with sensory and motor disabilities. In the survey 73% of the respondents rated or described their current health position as good to excellent. The Federal Health Department in Canada (Health and Welfare in Canada 1987) undertook a similar experiment and found the same results. These studies demonstrate quite convincingly that although disability is a factor, it is not the only determinant of whether or not a person feels healthy. These personal accounts of health and disability show that health care professionals ought to reconsider their perceptions and understanding of health and the way they go about providing health care. Furthermore it is interesting to note that when individuals interpret their disability as part of their life experiences then very often for them their disability ceases to be a handicap. Instead it becomes a challenge or an opportunity for creative growth and, paradoxically, a feeling of being alive (Hycner 1985, Lindsey 1996).

Resilience

Some people have the ability to adapt more successfully to adversity and disability than others. Many studies have investigated individuals who have managed to retain an optimism for life despite the existence of physical and psychological disability. Jacelon (1997) uses the word resilience to describe the specific trait that individuals exhibit in these circumstances. Resilience relates to the ability to spring back in the face of adversity. It also describes a personal characteristic that permits an individual to deal with the negative effects of stress and at the same time promote adaptation. Resilience is not a product but rather a process towards the restoration of homeostasis or balance. Therefore the promotion of resilience is dependent on the development of factors.

Fine (1991) found that personal perceptions and responses, particularly from other people, towards disability were crucial elements in the promotion of resilience. This study showed that, during the early stages, it was important for people with a physical disability to belong to a social group of people in the same position. They could take time to step back and view their position from the perspective of a spectator. This allowed them the space to experiment and attempt novel strategies at problem solving and adaptive behaviour and to recognise that there is more to oneself than the current circumstances would immediately suggest.

Resilience is a variable trait between individuals. There are, however, according to some studies, a number of predictors that suggest a greater potential for resilience. Resilient people usually have positive family support, are above average intelligence, have active and engaged lives and have a strong sense of self and self-reliance. The promotion of resilience should be of great interest to health care professionals. Nurses and others should be able to provide more appropriate and meaningful assistance for those people experiencing difficulties in coming to terms with their disability (Cowen & Work 1988, Jacelon 1997).

 Activities

- Carry out a brief literature review into the concept of health within disability in your library.
- Visit a patient with a disability that you have recently cared for and identify whether or not she feels healthy.

INDEPENDENT LIVING AND INCLUSIVENESS

Active members of the disabled community argue that recent care in the community legislation (NHS and Community Care Act 1990) limits the opportunity for disabled people to control their lives. The use of the term services for disabled people, they argue, needs to be extended and should conjure up ideas of support and acquire an enabling role, as for able-bodied

people. It has also been argued that services for disabled people should become commonplace. This is happening to an extent, for example audible pelican crossings, subtitles on television and sign language at public debates such as political party conferences. The sooner this becomes the norm across the spectrum of daily life, the sooner will be the full participation of disabled people.

Policies for the care of people with a disability now focus on a philosophy of equality and inclusiveness. New services are being developed that restate the civil rights of disabled people to work, housing and education. As a result they are contributing to a society that is now made richer from their contribution and disabled people are more organised and politically active in shedding the old and outdated paternalist ideas that predated this trend. Television and radio programmes produced and written by and for disabled people are now an accepted part of television planning (French 1994). When this level of communication and trust permeates throughout society, disabled people will begin to have an impact on the lives of able-bodied people in the same way that able-bodied people already influence disabled people (Batavia 1993).

DISABILITY AND THE LAW (Table 9.2)

The 1960s was a period of major political change in terms of empowering minority groups. Disabled groups began to align themselves together and form into a single minority group. In so doing they displayed a growing realisation that although there were differences in the nature of their disability and the individual effects, there were also underlying similarities. The most important of these were the core problems of poverty, discrimination and a lack of access to public services (including education, training and employment) that were freely accessible to able-bodied people. The Disabled Interest Group (DIG, formed in 1965 to organise a campaign for a special disability allowance for disabled people) was influential in pressurising the government to introduce the Chronically Sick and Disabled Person's Act 1970 (Wolfensberger 1989).

Table 9.2 Legislation for disabled people	
Act	Provisions
The Disabled Persons Employment Act 1944	Supported employment services for disabled people
The National Assistance Act 1948	Clear definition of disability
The Chronically Sick and Disabled Persons Act 1970	The provision of special services and support for disabled people

Disabled Persons Act

The Chronically Sick and Disabled Persons Act 1970 was designed to improve the support for disabled people living at home (Box 9.4). It placed a duty on local authorities to provide or assist with necessary help with needs such as adapting household facilities, the installation of a telephone and the provision of home care support. The legislation also made provision for the allocation of allowances to disabled people. This allowance, however, related closely to the level of dependency or restricted mobility. As a result it raised questions regarding fairness in the categorisations of disabled people. Miscalculations occurred because people obtained benefits following specific diagnoses rather than individual circumstances. The awarding of benefits ignored the degree of disability that existed and the level of restriction on the capacity to meet the daily living needs (Bond & Carstairs 1982, Duckworth 1983).

The Act was useful because it highlighted the needs of disabled people and included radical proposals for new services for disabled people. In spite of this it was criticised by disabled groups because it did little in terms of reducing

---

Box 9.4 Services for disabled people listed in the Chronically Sick and Disabled Persons Act 1970

Provision of practical assistance for the disabled person in the home
Assistance in the provision of television, telephone or recreational facilities
Provision of social and educational facilities outside of the home
Assistance in making necessary adaptations to the home to facilitate activities of daily living
Provision of meals either in or outside of the home

---

their continued segregation from the rest of society. They argued that the Act retained the idea that disability was the sole responsibility of the individual and nothing to do with the rest of society. In other words, able-bodied people were not expected to contribute in accommodating the needs of disabled people or assist in reducing discrimination.

Pressure continued to increase for further legislation that would affect the able-bodied community and in so doing substantially reduce the segregation mentality that existed. The rejuvenated disability movement that had its roots in the USA specifically wanted an end to the patronising attitude of the general public that was most obvious in television and radio programmes, certain films and newspapers. The aim was that a new spirit of inclusiveness should replace the marginalisation strategy. Disabled people expressed a demand for respect as thinking, politically aware people who could contribute in a rapidly changing technological world.

Activity

Discuss why disability groups displayed a reserved support for the Disabled Persons Act 1970.

Antidiscrimination legislation

The first attempts at putting antidiscrimination legislation against disabled people on to statute began about 1979. The Committee on Restrictions Against Disabled People considered a range of societal factors that created barriers for disabled people. The first of the report's 42 recommendations proposed that there should be legislation making discrimination illegal and that this should encompass every aspect of society (education, employment, transport and services). The delay in the publication of the report coincided with a change in government. As a result the issue was shelved, in spite of the fact that 1981 was set aside as an International Year for Disabled People, in which people with a disability were supposed to receive a special focus in terms of government policy.

Nevertheless the momentum and pressure for change in the law increased and eventually resulted in the passing of Disability Discrimination Act 1995. The government recognised that disabled people were discriminated against in that they received different treatment to other people, particularly in areas such as housing, training, education and employment (see Box 9.5). Frequently the cause of this discrimination was related to either prejudice or a failure by those in authority to discuss the matter with the disabled person. It was simply assumed that an individual could not carry out a particular task or use a particular service.

The Disability Discrimination Act 1995 began by redefining disability as a physical or mental impairment that has a substantial and long term adverse effect on a person's ability to carry out normal day-to-day activities. The Act applies to people with a substantial and long term physical, sensory or emotional disability. Severe disfigurement is also classed as a disability. People who have a disability and people who have had a disability in the past but no longer have one are both covered by the Act. An example of this second group could be people who have in the past suffered from epilepsy.

There are a few circumstances in which it is not possible to treat disabled people as favourably as others (see also Table 9.3). They include circumstances of either health and safety or where a person cannot understand the nature of a contract because of their disability. If, however, it is proven that the person is not a health or safety risk or does appreciate the nature of a contract then it is considered to be illegal if they are treated differently. The law does not prevent disabled people being treated more favourably in certain circumstances. For example if a professional football club wished to provide sideline positions for wheelchair bound people it would be able to do so. Similarly, cinema owners may continue to offer hearing impaired people front stall seats at the same price as more expensive seats in other parts of the building.

Box 9.5 Discrimination and the law

Under the law discrimination is said to occur when:

- a disabled person is treated less favourably than someone else
- the different treatment is for a reason relating to the person's disability
- there is no legitimate justification for different treatment
- there is a failure to make a reasonable adjustment for a disabled person

The rights of disabled people

The Disability Discrimination Act brought in new rules that aim to end the discrimination that many disabled people have faced in the past. The Act gives disabled people new rights in the areas of employment, accessing services and buying or renting land or property. The Act requires schools, colleges and universities to provide specific information for disabled people. It allows the government to set minimum

Table 9.3 Employment	
Adjustments made by employers	Example
Altering premises	Doors may be widened or special WC facilities may be installed
Minor duties	A person with a hearing deficit may not have to answer the telephone if an adjustment to the telephone isn't satisfactory to the disabled person

standards so that disabled people can use public transport more easily. In addition, it requires the setting up of a National Disability Council to advise the government on the need for policy changes or of any potential for discrimination against disabled people.

The law places a significant responsibility on employers. Following the implementation of the Disability Discrimination Act, it will be illegal to treat a disabled person less favourably than someone else because of their disability, without good reason. This applies to all aspects of employment matters, including selection, interviewing, recruitment, training, promotion and dismissal. Furthermore, employers must look at and make changes that could possibly affect the potential recruitment of an individual with a disability. In so doing it is argued that the employer will be able to recruit the best person for the job irrespective of the presence of any form of disability. The law also signalled the end of disabled people registering their disability and the quota system that previously existed.

The law affects anyone who provides any goods or service to the general public. This could range from buying a drink in a pub, eating out in a restaurant or doing the weekly shopping in the supermarket. It will be against the law to refuse to serve anyone because of their disability. It will also be illegal to offer a disabled person a service that is not of the same standard as would be offered to everyone else. For example it will be unlawful to ask someone with a hearing problem or disfigurement to sit in a special place in a restaurant. The government anticipates that in time all disabled people will have full access to all forms of public transport. This will include buses, coaches, trains and aeroplanes. The government believes that, for example, all people who use wheelchairs will be able to hire a taxi in the street or at a rank, the same as everybody else.

DISABILITY COUNCIL

The National Disability Council (or in Northern Ireland the Northern Ireland Disability Council) is responsible for advising the government on all issues related to the employment and training of disabled people. The main objective of the council is to eliminate and reduce the incidence of discrimination against disabled people. The council also has a monitoring role in terms of the full implementation of the Act and will have to produce a report each year. The report, which will go before parliament, will outline the activities it has engaged in throughout the preceding year. The council is also expected to advise the government on the need for further policy change if this is necessary. Before advising the government they will be expected to have carried out an audit and costing of the net effects of implementing their advice. In addition they should have consulted with other relevant bodies that have an interest in the matter that is being proposed. The council is composed of between 10 and 20 members appointed by the Secretary of State for Social Security. The membership must either appreciate the needs of disabled people; have a disability; or have experience of business, industry or the professions.

Activities

- List the five main features of the Disability Discrimination Act.
- Discuss with your colleagues what the cumulative effect will be for people with a disability.
- Organise a debate with your colleagues regarding the need for the Disability Discrimination Act.

Conclusion

Most curricula for health care professionals have expanded to be more inclusive of diverse elements in society. Some of the more common themes pursued by undergraduate programmes address the experiences of different countries' health and social care services; the experiences of women; ethnic problems and racial problems. Disability debates rarely achieve the same degree of intensity as these, even though there are far more people with a disability and more diverse needs than other minorities. Some specialised public policy programmes mention disability in the context of health issues, or education, or long term care for the elderly for example. They do not, however, consider disability in the context of civil rights nor do they address the spectrum of need between, for example, those people with physical or learning disabilities. The National Health Service and Community Care Act 1990 has proved to be a window of opportunity for some disabled people. According to the Act, money for services should follow patients and services should be provided as a response to an identified need. The independent living scheme has taken this idea one step further in terms of maximising the empowerment of disabled people. This scheme allows the disabled person to take control of advertising, recruiting and interviewing personal assistants. Money

does not go directly to the disabled person but for all practical purposes the disabled person is assuming the role of employer. This has a significant effect in reducing the professional influence over the disabled person as well as within the specific relationship with the personal assistant (Fowler et al 1996).

Activities

- Discuss with your colleagues what more can be done to enable people with a disability to become fully integrated members of society.
- Select any public facility that you use (your campus, for example, or a local hospital) and list some of the factors that make it more and less accessible for people with a disability.

REFERENCES

Barnes C 1992 Disabling imagery and the media: the British Council of Organisations of Disabled People. Ryburn, Halifax

Batavia A I 1993 Relating disability policy to broader public policy. Policy Studies Journal 21(4):735–739

Blaxter M 1980 The meaning of disability, 2nd edn. Heinemann, London

Bond J, Carstairs V 1982 Services for the elderly. Scottish Health Services Studies No. 42. Scottish Home and Health Department, Edinburgh

Cowen E L, Work W C 1988 Resilient children, psychological wellness and primary prevention. American Journal of Community Psychology 16(4):591–607

Davidhizar R 1997 Disability does not have to be the grief that never ends: helping patients adjust. Rehabilitation Nursing 22(1):32–35

Davis K 1996 Disability and legislation: rights and equality. In: Hales G (ed) Beyond disability towards an enabling society. Sage, London

Duckworth D 1983 The classification and measurement of disablement. Research Report No. 10. DHSS Social Research Branch/HMSO, London

Fowler B, Carrivick P, Carrello J, McFarlane C 1996 The rehabilitation success rate: an organizational performance. International Journal of Rehabilitation and Research 19(4):341–343

Fine S B 1991 Resilience and human adaptability: who rises above adversity. American Journal of Occupational Therapy 45(6): 493–503. Cited in: Jacelon CS 1997 The trait and process of resilience. Journal of Advanced Nursing 25:123–129

Fox R C 1990 Training in caring competence in North America. Humane Medicine 6(1):15–21

French S 1994 On equal terms: working with disabled people. Butterworth Heinemann, London

Goffman E 1984 Notes on the management of spoiled identity. Pelican, London

Hales G (ed) 1996 Beyond disability towards an enabling society. Sage, London

Hahn H 1993 The potential impact of disability studies on political science (as well as vice-versa). Policy Studies Journal 21(4):740–751

Health and Welfare in Canada 1987 The active health report: perspectives on Canada's health promotion survey: Minister of Supply and Services, Ottawa

Hycner R H 1985 Some guidelines for the phenomenological analysis of interview data. Human Studies 8(3):279–303

Illich I 1976 Medical nemesis: the expropriation of health. Random, New York

Jacelon C S 1997 The trait and process of resilience. Journal of Advanced Nursing 25:123–129

Lindsey E 1996 Health within illness: experiences of chronically ill/disabled people. Journal of Advanced Nursing 24:465–472

Moch S D 1989 Health within illness: conceptual evolution and practice possibilities. Advances in Nursing Science 11(4):23–31

Morris J 1993 Independent lives?: community care and disabled people. Macmillan, London

Oliver M 1996 Understanding disability from theory to practice. Macmillan, London

Orem D 1991 Nursing: concepts of practice, 4th edn. Mosby, London

Parse R R 1990 Health: a personal commitment. Nursing Science Quarterly 3:136–140

Pender N 1990 Expressing health through lifestyle patterns. Nursing Science Quarterly 3:115–122

Pfeiffer D 1993 Overview of the disability movement:

history, legislative record and political implications. Policy Studies Journal 21(4):724–734

Redman B K 1993 The process of patient education. Mosby, London

Rodgers S, Marini I 1994 Physiological and psychological aspects of aging with spinal cord injury. Scientific Psychosocial Processes 7(3):98–103

Scott-Parker 1989 They aren't in the brief. King's Fund Centre, London

Smith B 1996 Working choices. In: Hales G (ed) Beyond disability towards an enabling society. Sage, London

Stuifbergen A K, Becker H A, Ingalsbe K, Sands D 1990 Perception of health among adults with disabilities. Health Values 14(2):18–26

Szymanski E M, Trueba H T 1994 Castification of people with disabilities: potential disempowering aspects of classification in disability services. Journal of Rehabilitation 60(3):12–20

Tannahill A 1990 Health education and promotion: planning for the 1990s. Health Education Journal 49(4):194–197

Theuerkauf S, Carpenter P 1992 Return to the real world: a spinal cord injury. Journal of Home Health Care Practice 4(4):14–23

Thorne S 1993 Negotiating health care: the social context of chronic illness. Sage, Newbury Park, California

Titmuss R 1963 Essays on the welfare state. Unwin, London

Townsend P, Davidson N 1982 Inequalities and health: the Black Report. Harmondsworth, London

Twigg J 1997 Deconstructing the social bath: help with bathing at home for older and disabled people. Journal of Social Policy 26(2):193–210

Union of the Physically Impaired Against Segregation 1976 Fundamental principles of disability. UPIAS, London

Watson S D 1993 Introduction: disability policy as an emerging field of mainstream public policy research and pedagogy. Policy Studies Journal 21(4):720–723

WHO 1980 International classification of impairment, disabilities and handicaps. WHO, Geneva

Wolfensberger W 1989 Human service policies: the rhetoric versus the reality. In: Barton L (ed) Disability and dependence. Falmer, London

Learning disabilities and mental health

Owen Barr

10

At the end of the chapter the student will be able to:

- **outline the evolution of hospital and community services for people with learning disabilities and mental illness**
- **explore the changing social and political factors that have shaped services over the past 50 years**
- **evaluate the degree to which current services have realised the anticipated goals of community care**
- **evaluate the impact of social policy/service changes on the life of people with learning disabilities and mental illness**
- **discuss the possible shape of future services and what implications this may have for clients, families and professionals.**

Introduction

Despite the obvious differences, there are many similarities in the way that services for people with learning disabilities and people with mental health needs have emerged. Often new legislation introduced and reports specifically commissioned to review services have simultaneously considered the abilities and needs of both client groups. This is in part a product of history and the longstanding association between services for people with learning disabilities and people with mental health needs. The association in recent times does appear to be gradually reducing and this is reflected in the increasing number of specifically focused social policy developments that attempt to make recommendations for discrete groups of people.

Following a brief historical overview of the development of services prior to the 1954 Royal Commission, this chapter will focus on key changes in social policy and service principles that relate to people with learning disabilities and people with mental illness and their influence on services. It will also identify how social policy changes that focused on children have reshaped some aspects of services for children with learning disabilities and mental health needs. It will draw mainly from the legislation which applies to England and Wales. A summary of this, and of legislation for Scotland and Northern Ireland, is presented in Table 10.1.

DEFINING THE TERMS

A variety of current legal definitions (at times inconsistent with each other) relate to people with learning disabilities; they include mental impairment, severe mental impairment, and (in Northern Ireland) mental handicap, severe mental handicap and severe mental impairment (Box 10.1). The term 'people with learning disabilities' was introduced in 1990 as a replacement term for 'people with a mental handicap'. 'People with learning disabilities' appears to be the most widely accepted expression at present and will be used in this chapter, although at times other terms may be used for accuracy when referring to historical facts or literature.

It is acknowledged that precise definitions are difficult when considering sensitive subjects such as learning disabilities, due to the variations in the abilities and needs of those people it involves. The purpose of definitions is primarily for administrative or legal reasons. Other, psychological based, definitions relating to people with learning disabilities have been developed, but have not been found to be entirely satisfactory either (Burton 1997).

Despite apparent inconsistencies, some key aspects of definitions of people with learning disabilities and people with mental health needs do exist. There is a general consensus that

Table 10.1 Overview of some key legislation relating to people with learning disabilities, people with mental illness and children from 1959 to March 1998. It is important to be aware of legislation specific to the country in which you are working as sections often differ, as can some powers within the legislation. It is also important in academic work to use correct references. (*March 1998.*)

England & Wales	Scotland	N. Ireland
1959 Mental Health	1960 Mental Health (Scotland) Act	1961 Mental Health Act
1971 Education Act	1969 Education (Scotland) Act	No corresponding legislation
1981 Education Act	1980 Education (Scotland) Act	1986 Education & Libraries Order
1983 Mental Health Act	1984 Mental Health (Scotland) Act	1986 Mental Health Order
1989 Children's Act	1995 Children's (Scotland) Act	1995 Children's (NI) Order
1990 NHS & Community Care Act	1990 NHS & Community Care Act (Specific section for Scotland)	1991 Personal Health & Social Services Order
1995 Carers (Recognition & Services) Act	1995 Carers (Recognition & Services) Act (Specific section for Scotland)	No corresponding legislation to be introduced. Operates as 'good practice'. No legal right to assessment
1996 Disability Discrimination Act	1996 Disability Discrimination Act (Specific section for Scotland)	No corresponding legislation (at present). Race Relations Order introduced in 1997. This was the equivalent to the 1976 Race Relations Act (England & Wales)
1996 Mental Health (Patients in the Community) Act	1996 Mental Health (Patients in the Community) Act (Specific section for Scotland)	No corresponding legislation (at present)
1996 Direct Care Payments. Care in the Community Act.	1996 Direct Care Payments. Care in Community Act	No corresponding legislation (at present)

Box 10.1 Various current legal definitions

Mental impairment: A state of arrested or incomplete development of mind which includes significant impairment of intelligence and social functioning (England & Wales).

Mental handicap: A state of arrested or incomplete development of mind which includes significant impairment of intelligence and social functioning (N. Ireland).

Severe mental handicap: A state of arrested or incomplete development of mind which includes severe impairment of intelligence and social functioning.

Severe mental impairment: A state of arrested or incomplete development of mind which includes severe impairment of intelligence and social functioning associated with abnormally aggressive or seriously irresponsible conduct.

Mental illness: A state of mind which affects a person's thinking, perceiving, emotion or judgement to an extent that he requires care or medical treatment in his own interests or in the interests of other persons.

learning disabilities involve a degree of impairment of intelligence and social functioning, and that the condition presents during childhood and is relatively permanent. Learning disability does not normally involve aggressive behaviour and this has been reflected by defining people with abnormally aggressive behaviour as having a mental impairment or severe mental impairment. In the UK difficulties in learning, such as dyslexia or attention deficit disorder, are also excluded.

Activities

- Working as a group of 4–6 students, compile a list of terms you have heard people with learning disabilities and people with mental illness referred to by.
- Discuss the origins and relative merits of each term as a group, providing an explanation as to the reasons why you feel the way you do.
- As a group, write a list of what you think are the positive and negative implications of using 'labels' for groups of people.
- Prepare in your own words definitions for people with learning disabilities and people with mental illness, and a list of criteria for the appropriate use of the definitions.

HISTORICAL DEVELOPMENT OF SERVICES

Historical accounts of the care of people with learning disabilities reveal a wide range of responses, varying from treating them as special people who should be respected and well looked after to evidence that the care of people with learning disabilities and people with mental illness was sometimes characterised by abuse, ill treatment, an association with witchcraft and possible infanticide. (Key developments prior to 1904 are outlined in Box 10.2. For further historical information see Atkinson et al 1997, Rogers & Pilgrim 1996, Wright & Digby 1996.)

Box 10.2 Key dates in the development of services prior to 1904

1325 The 'De Praerogative Regis' provided some early guidelines about how the property of lunatics and idiots should be looked after, although this was not statute (Neugebauer 1996)

1377 Bethlehem Hospital opened in London

1625 The Land Act distinguished between idiots and lunatics, enabling the king to have land inherited by such people on a temporary or permanent basis

1736 Abolition of laws against witchcraft

1744 The separation of lunatics, vagrants and paupers

1763 Attempts to regulate 'madhouses'. People paid an entrance fee and many visited to look at and taunt people in hospital

1801 Itard's work with the 'Wild boy of Averyon' demonstrating that people with learning disabilities could learn new skills

1828 and 1853 Increased the degree of structure and regulation of the lunatic asylums

Mid-1800s 'Colonies for mental defectives' started to emerge

1860s Francis Galton was a key figure in the Eugenics movement. There were also moves towards segregated services to protect society (although the Eugenics Education Society wasn't formally set up until 1907)

1886 The Idiots Act: highlighted a duty to care for people under the Act and put asylums under the control of local county councils

1890 The Lunacy Act: defined an insane person as an idiot, lunatic or person of unsound mind. Despite the considerable progress that was made, it is clear that the level of understanding remained limited (Neugebauer 1996)

The consolidation of segregated services, 1904–1950

A Royal Commission in 1904 emphasised the importance of protecting people from society, and recommended that all people with learning disabilities and mental illness should be identified, registered and put in touch with caring services. It also recommended that local networks of services should be coordinated through a central body. The report of this Royal Commission also formed the basis for the 1913 Mental Deficiency Act. The Mental Deficiency Act also signalled the emergence of a medical model for care and the medicalisation of people with learning disabilities and people with mental illness. The reasons for this relate to doctors assuming an increased role in this specific service and the fact that medical treatment became a key focus in the provision of services.

The Mental Health Treatment Act 1930 introduced the terms 'voluntary' and 'detained' status for patients. Before this all admissions to hospital were compulsory with limited avenues for appeal. Also at this time, clear legal differences were introduced separating people with learning disabilities from people with a mental illness. In spite of the introduction of a clear boundary, it appears that provision for people with learning disabilities continued to be within the broader category of 'mental health' services.

The 1944 Education Act was the first Education Act of major significance for people with learning disabilities. The Act acknowledged the need to provide education to some people with learning disabilities up to the age of 16 years. In spite of a growing awareness of the nature of learning disabilities, this legislation relied solely on intelligence tests to decide who could benefit from education. This rather crude strategy classified those people with an IQ between 50 and 70 as educationally subnormal. Those with an IQ below 50, who it was erroneously believed could not benefit from education, were classified as ineducable. The net effect was the exclusion of all people with an IQ of less than 50 from appropriate statutory education provision, a position that remained unchanged until 1971 in Britain, and 1986 in Northern Ireland.

A NEW ERA

The next major change in the development of current service for people with learning disabilities and people with mental illness was the introduction of the National Health Services Act in 1948. This resulted in former 'colonies' (by this time referred to as hospitals as a result of changes within the Mental Treatment Act 1930 (Gladden 1997)) being taken under the control of the National Health Service. A key consequence of the Second World War and the subsequent investigations that followed raised the profile of people with a learning disability as an issue of human rights. This resulted in the Universal Declaration of Human Rights (United Nations 1948) and the European Convention on Human Rights (Council of Europe 1950 – only accepted into UK law in 1997). The focus of attention on human rights issues had major consequences for people with learning disabilities as well as people with mental illness, particularly as a deterrent to the Eugenics movement. (Although the movement had been in decline since the mid 1920s, this international focus certainly speeded up the process.)

In the UK, a Royal Commission on Law relating to Mental Illness and Mental Deficiency published a report, in 1957, that formed the basis for the review of the next mental health legislation (the Mental Health Act 1959). Significant changes to the principles of the mental health legislation were introduced, several of which were instrumental in shaping services that currently exist. Definitions relating to people with learning disabilities were amended and the terms mental subnormality and severe mental subnormality were introduced to replace idiot, imbecile, feeble minded and moral defective. However, these definitions continued to based on intelligence and no clear account was taken of the levels of an individual's social functioning.

The 1959 Act also developed ideas such as voluntary admissions and the rights of people compulsorily detained and admitted to hospital.

People compulsorily detained in hospital were afforded the right to have their status reviewed regularly by a new body called the Mental Health Review Tribunal. This body had the authority to rescind compulsory admissions and detentions of people in hospital. Local authorities were given a statutory responsibility to provide community based services for people with learning disabilities and people with a mental illness. This was one of the earliest steps toward the development of care in the community for these two groups. However, progress towards community based services was slow.

During the 1960s many 'hostels' were opened during this first phase. However, as Race (1995) points out, although local authorities were statutorily obliged to provide residential and day care services in the community, the funding and provision of hospitals remained under the control of the health service. It is suggested that, as a consequence, local authorities focused on the development of day care as opposed to residential care facilities, including adult and 'junior training centres'. These latter were for children with learning disabilities who continued to be classed as 'ineducable'. Despite the considerable policy changes brought about by the Mental Health Act, services continued to receive criticism because of their reliance on large hospitals as the focus for service provision for this group. Because of this, a medical model for providing care remained the philosophical underpinning for services.

It is accepted that important medical developments of great value were made during this period, such as the introduction of neuroleptic medicines that can be used to suppress symptoms of some mental illnesses and some behaviour difficulties among people with learning disabilities. Discoveries were also made regarding the causation of some conditions that lead to the development of learning disabilities (Gilbert 1993). Although the medical model of services was probably at its strongest at this time, new educational and social models were beginning to gain influence and create pressure to move services in a new and creative direction.

The need for hospitals services?

During the 1950s an expanding body of knowledge began to question whether or not large hospitals were suitable places for the provision of effective care and treatment. The origin of this debate arose from three sources. First, there was growing evidence that people with learning disabilities were able to learn new skills and that many could become self-supporting. This work focused particularly on teaching repetitive light industrial tasks and found that these could be learned gradually, in steps. These findings were a significant influence in the organisation of work in adult training centre workshops. The evidence that people with learning disabilities could be educated and make an economic contribution to society seriously challenged the long-held belief that education for them was of limited value (Race 1995). In many ways, the period between the early 1950s and the late 1960s saw a re-emergence of an optimism about the abilities of people which had been dormant since the mid-1800s.

Second, research studies highlighted the negative impact of the hospital environment on the behaviour and achievements of patients (see Race 1995 for a detailed summary of the 1950–1960 major research findings). Barton (1959) and Goffman (1961) in particular were major contributors in this area. Barton went as far as describing a condition referred to as 'institutional neurosis' that was attributable to the rigidity, isolation and loss of prospects of the total hospital environment, an environment that retained a custodial approach and required passivity among patients. The process of institutionalisation affected the behaviour, abilities and social world of all people within it, including the staff. Its effects included apathy, lack of initiative, apparent inability to make plans for the future and a lack of individuality (Barton 1976). In addition, the structural design of the majority of hospitals for people with learning disabilities and people with mental illness in the 1950s and 1960s promoted segregation of those in hospital from the rest of society and therefore encouraged institutionalisation.

Thirdly, there was increasing concern over the degree of protection for people in hospital. Reports of wrongful detentions were not uncommon and, coupled with the information about institutionalisation, evidence of mistreatment, cruelty and exploitation was increasing. The evidence showed that hospitals were socially isolated, focused on containment, lacked a positive rehabilitative orientation and provided a fragmented service with poor communication among professions. This culminated in a series of reports following enquiries in many hospitals, such as Ely Hospital (1969), Whittingham Hospital (1972), South Ockenden Hospital (1974) and Normansfield Hospital (1978).

Activities

Obtain a copy of any of the enquiries listed, and any new inquiries into your local services:

- Identify five significant findings of the enquiries and provide an explanation as to why you think those identified are the most important.
- From the significant findings identified, make a list of any indications of these findings that may exist in your services.
- Identify five actions you can take to maintain your own professional practice, discuss these with group members and your lecturer and put them into action.

NORMALISATION – A REVISION OF SERVICE PRINCIPLES

Although the philosophy of 'normalisation' began in Scandinavian countries in the 1950s, it was the late 1960s before it had a significant impact on social policy in the UK. In spite of this late start, it has remained the major guiding philosophy for services ever since (Brown & Smith 1992). The core of normalisation is asserting the rights of people and the need to accept everybody as an individual. Normalisation emphasises the need to 'use means which are valued in our society, in order to develop and support personal characteristics, behaviours and experiences which are likewise valued'. In essence, it is about 'revaluing devalued people' (Tyne & O'Brien 1981).

The principles within normalisation were in contrast to the previous custodial and segregation based approaches to services. It rejected the need for control over clients, and highlighted a need to work with people in order that they could become socially valued and integrated into local communities. Services that incorporate normalisation in practice should be characterised by particular attributes (O'Brien 1992). Clients should have opportunities to become involved in ordinary activities like other members of society. Individuals should be facilitated to actively participate in decisions about their daily activities and any decisions that affect them. Real choice between socially valued options should be an integral part of services. This should involve respecting individuals as valued people irrespective of their physical or cognitive ability. Normalisation also requires a more accepting and valuing attitude towards people with learning disabilities and people with mental illness among members of the public (Barr 1995).

Education

The 1971 Education Act (England & Wales) removed the category of 'ineducable' previously attached to people with an IQ below 50. All children became entitled to access to education up to the age of 16 and were permitted to stay on until the age of 19. Consistent with a new emphasis towards education, the responsibility for providing schools for people with learning disabilities was transferred from social services departments to the local education authorities on 1 April 1971. In Northern Ireland the transfer took place at a later date, principally because of the differences in administration. It was argued that the transfer of responsibility would create opportunities for real benefits for children with learning disabilities through the availability of educational advice, comprehensive professional training for staff, increased flexibility in placing children and the emphasis on social adaptation, language development and the development of socially acceptable behaviour (DHSS 1971). Local education authorities were also responsible for the education of children in hospital.

However, integrated nursery and playgroups services for children with disabilities remained the responsibility of social services departments.

Inclusiveness

The emphasis of the new services clearly focused on reducing segregation and incorporated the principles of normalisation. It was argued that changes in 'labels' and terminology were important in reducing segregation and the term 'mental handicap' was introduced in 1971 as an agreed preference. It was believed that it emphasised a renewed attitude to negative labels that would be equally applicable to other forms of handicap, that is to 'prevent it whenever possible, to assess it adequately when it occurs, and to do everything possible to alleviate its severity and compensate for its effects' (DHSS 1971, p. 1).

The utilisation of mainstream facilities was another key strategy in reducing the segregation of people with learning disabilities and people with mental illness in local communities. All new buildings had to be close to the communities they served, unlike many of the existing hospitals, which were considerable distances away from centres of population. All residential developments were required to have a community orientation and incorporate a 'homelike' environment. Residential accommodation hostels should no longer be so impersonal, but must become more like homes for the inhabitants. It was also recommended that the maximum size of hostels should be limited to 25 places for adults and 20 for children. Hospitals too were expected to become more homelike, and to remove their previous custodial and unstimulating environments.

It was anticipated that, in the future, people requiring residential accommodation would live in community-based units and that hospitals admissions would be reserved for those people requiring either treatment or constant supervision. Hospitals were no longer to be used as places of long term residential accommodation (DHSS 1971). Clear targets were set to reduce the numbers of hospital beds for people with learning disabilities (DHSS 1971) and people

with mental illness (DHSS 1975). The continued reliance on hospital services was a major criticism of the vision of services in the 1970s. The Jay Report (DHSS 1979) argued that, in services for people with learning disabilities, progress could only be made by radical changes in how services were organised and delivered. These radical changes involved a predominant shift to a social model of care, hospital closures, and stopping specialist pre-registration nurse education for nurses of people with learning disabilities in favour of further developing social work courses in residential care. The social model of services and the rights of people with learning disabilities presented in the Jay Report (see Box 10.3) became the benchmark for services emerging in the 1980s and were mirrored in services for people with mental illness.

Coordination of service planning

Joint planning between health and social service authorities became a key feature of the 1970s within progressive mental health and learning disability services. This process evolved to incorporate also voluntary sector agencies. Several reports during the 1970s called for additional resources for service developments (DHSS 1971, 1975, 1979). Although some additional funds were made available to encourage joint planning, a consistent theme of government documents during the 1970s was that much more could be achieved by increased efficiency in the management of available resources. No clear decision was noted in policy documents during the 1970s about a need for a lead agency in coordinating community based services. However, the main thrust of emerging documents identified this need for the achievement of social models of care. To assist in achieving this objective a National Development Group (NDG) and National Development Team (NDT) were set up in 1975. These consisted of health and social care professionals, legal representatives and lay people. Their purpose was to advise government regarding the continued development and implementation of service policies for people with learning disabilities (NDG 1977, NDT 1978).

Box 10.3 Principles of services for people with learning disabilities as outlined in the Jay Report (1979)

- Mentally handicapped people have a right to enjoy normal patterns of life within the community.
- Mentally handicapped people will have a right to be treated as individuals.
- Mentally handicapped people will require additional help from communities in which they live, and from professional services, if they are to develop to the maximum potential as individuals.
- Mentally handicapped children should be able to live with a family. The first question to be asked must always be 'How can we provide support which will allow the child to continue to live with his own parents and his own brothers and sisters, in his own home, in his own community?'. If this proves impossible, we must look first to a long term placement with a substitute family.
- Any mentally handicapped adult who wishes to leave his or her parental home should have the opportunity to do so.
- Any accommodation provided for adults or children should allow the individual to live as a member of a small group.
- If they so wish, mentally handicapped people should be able to live with their peers who are not mentally handicapped. The corollary is that non-handicapped members of the community have a right to grow up and learn to live with their less able fellow citizens.
- Staffed accommodation should, wherever possible, be provided in suitably adapted houses which are physically integrated with the community.
- These homes should be as local as possible to help the handicapped person to retain contact with his own family and community. This means that we need a highly dispersed system of homes. Clustering a number of living units together, whilst it might still allow small group living, would inevitably infringe this principle of locality (or localness).
- Mentally handicapped people should be able to live in a mixed sex environment. For adults this would include the right and opportunities to get married.
- Mentally handicapped people should be able to develop a daily routine like other people.

In practice these principles involve developing services which ensure:

- There should be a proper separation of home, work and recreation.
- The right of an individual to live, learn and work in the least restrictive environment appropriate to that particular person.
- The right to make or be involved in decisions that affect oneself.
- Acceptance that individual needs differ not only between different handicapped individuals, but within the same individual over time.
- The right of parents to be involved in decisions about their children.

The needs of 'families' and children

Prior to the 1970s little attention was given at policy level to assisting the families of people with learning disabilities and people with mental illness. The overriding utilitarian attitude prevailed that families should be responsible for their own members. When families could no longer cope the only alternative for the person was a place in 'permanent' residential care, which in effect usually meant a large hospital far away from his home. Difficulties in maintaining active family contact from these hospitals were often compounded by failing health of parents, a sense of failure in parents and other family members and rigidity in hospital routines.

The growing body of research knowledge into the impact of people with learning disabilities (Barr 1996) and people with mental illness in the family highlighted the need to increase support to families if admissions to hospital were to be reduced. For the first time families became recognised as cohesive units that needed a co-ordinated response. There was a growing move away from treating only the person with learning disabilities or the person with mental illness and the avoidance of family difficulties that frequently impinged on their ability to continue to provide care. The possibility that families and family environments may be triggers for the development of mental difficulties in children was also recognised as needing specific attention (DHSS 1975).

During the 1970s children with learning disabilities or mental illness emerged as a separate entity within services for the first time (DHSS 1971, 1975, 1976, 1978, 1979). Up until the 1970s services made little distinction between the needs of children and adults in hospitals. This resulted in major reform of residential accommodation. This revised attitude was clearly evident in the Court Report (DHSS 1976) which stated that: 'severely mentally handicapped children have more in common with other children because of their childhood, than they do with severely mentally handicapped adults because of their common disability'.

This view was further expanded by the NDG

into a principle of service planning: 'children are children first and mentally handicapped second' (NDG 1977, p. 2). The NDG pamphlet, *Mentally handicapped children: a plan for action* (NDG 1977), consolidated a vision of future services for children and their families and the ideas introduced then form the basis of many current services. The Court Report gave specific attention to the needs of children with mental illness and highlighted the need to recognise their childhood. It also recommended setting up child development clinics and child surveillance programmes to monitor the progress of the child with additional needs. It was proposed that a district handicap team, responsible for all children with disabilities, would be the most effective way to coordinate services to children.

A variety of measures were put in place during the 1970s to increase the practical support for families. These included the introduction of Attendance Allowance, the provision of local community based respite care, increased home help support, the introduction of laundry support, an additional emphasis on making nursery and playgroup places available for children with learning disabilities and the requirement to complete a comprehensive multidisciplinary assessment of family abilities and needs. Further to this, the right of parents to be more actively involved in influencing decisions affecting their children was recognised (in good practice but not in law) and there was greater availability of information for parents to assist in decision making.

Professional staff were also encouraged to work in collaboration with parents to facilitate the development of parental support networks. There were developments in the provision of emergency support, out-patient clinics, day care and day hospitals, and domiciliary support from the increasing number of community learning disability teams (Hall & Russell 1985) and community mental health teams. In addition, the right of a person with learning disabilities to leave their parental home as part of the normal development (and not due to crisis intervention) was an important recommendation from the Jay Report (DHSS 1979).

Activities

- Obtain a copy of *Helping mentally handicapped people in hospital* (NDG 1978) for a vision of new hospital services. Discuss with your colleagues how much change has come about in the interim period.
- Review the principles that were outlined in the Jay Report, and then:
  — during your placement in clinical setting for people with learning disabilities, identify any evidence that exists to demonstrate how these principles have been implemented within your services.
  — list any principles for which evidence of implementation cannot be found and discuss with colleagues why this may be so.
  — outline action that you may take within your personal sphere of responsibility to work towards the principles identified as absent.

Substantive change in the 1970s?

There is little doubt that the developments towards the vision of community based services and a shift from hospital services outlined during the 1970s formed the foundation of current and developing services. However, it appears that progress towards community based services was limited. Evidence of patchy progress towards meeting the 1971 recommendations for people with learning disabilities was noted by both the National Development Group (NDG 1977) and the Jay Report (DHSS 1979). In 1975 community services for people with mental illness were described as a 'comparative rarity' (DHSS 1975).

Many of the ideas set out then remain challenges in practice now, such as the successful rundown of hospitals, the development of multidisciplinary team work, and the increased accountability of individual practitioners and service managers. The suggested rapid pace of change together with the shift to social services and the uncertainty that this created, and the reduced acknowledgement of the positive contribution of health services were compounded by the overlaps and struggles to assert new professional roles. These factors did result in a degree of discontent among members of multidisciplinary teams (Rose 1993).

MENTAL HEALTH COMMISSION

The Mental Health Act 1983 (England & Wales) and equivalent legislation for Northern Ireland and Scotland required the setting up of a new body called the Mental Health Commission (consisting of lay people, lawyers, voluntary group representatives, and health and social care professionals) to monitor the care of people with mental illness and people with learning disabilities. Clients and members of the public can have direct access to members of the Commission to discuss aspects of individual care or wider service issues. It is also important to note that this legislation increased the frequency of possible appeals by people detained in hospital to the Mental Health Review Tribunal. The need to register people with learning disabilities was removed by this legislation (only to be reintroduced for children within a few years). It also excluded from the definition of mental disorder people with problems with personality disorder, promiscuity or other immoral conduct, sexual deviancy and dependence on alcohol or drugs. Definitions of people with learning disabilities were amended to incorporate 'an impairment of intelligence and social functioning', thereby recognising the limitations of intelligence as the only measure.

COMMUNITY CARE

The examination of hospitals as the focus of services that commenced during the 1960s continued with some vigour into the 1970s. After a considerable period of inattention, the plight of people in hospitals was highlighted in the media and became a major political issue. It was against this backdrop of increasing dissatisfaction and heightened public concern that the government published two documents. One outlined a vision of 'better services' for people with learning disabilities (DHSS 1971) and the other addressed the needs of people with mental health problems (DHSS 1975).

These documents included a reaffirmation of several of the priorities contained in the earlier Royal Commission (1954–1957), as well as presenting new ideas for services that provided a clear picture of the government's priorities for future development. Perhaps the most profound change arising in the 1970s was a confirmation that all people have an ability to learn, and the belief that all people should have the opportunity to maximise their abilities and to develop new skills. Together with the renewed focus on rehabilitating people with mental illness there was evidence of a commitment at policy level to overturn the previous pessimistic dogma that characterised the custodial services of the 1950s and 1960s.

In the 1980s it was time to show that community care could work in practice. The decade was characterised by the scrutiny of developing services, challenges of progress to date and disagreements over the definition and practicalities of community care. Despite the raft of reports that were issued in the previous decade incorporating a community based approach, considerable debate and uncertainty existed about how best to put community care into practice.

Care by the community

Little empirical evidence existed to support the claims made for community care, but there was a firm belief that it would work. In essence a 'notional consensus' about the nature of community care existed (Wolfensberger & Thomas 1994), in that most people had a general understanding of the concept but varying and often conflicting ideas about how to put it into practice. Some debate arose about the differences between care in the community and care by the community. It was noted that although the 1970s vision was of care provided by a variety of agencies (mainly statutory) *in* the community, by the early 1980s the implementation was moving towards care *by* the community (McCarthy 1989).

Changing ideologies

The implications of this shift was that policy was no longer about the statutory agencies providing most services, but rather the community (the core and extended family, voluntary and private sector and local neighbourhoods) using more of its own resources. In recognition of the debate surrounding the nature of community care, some attempts were made to clarify the components. The Short Report defined it as 'a preference for home life over institutional care; a preference for the ideal of normalisation and integration and the avoidance so far as is possible of separate provision, segregation and restriction; a preference for small over large; and a preference for local services over distant ones' (DHSS 1985).

Further to the ideological debates, evidence was emerging that progress towards community care for people with learning disabilities was 'disappointingly slow'. The limited progress that existed was patchy and impaired by confusion over the roles and responsibilities of individual staff and their respective agencies. It was also noted that spending on hospitals remained high and long term admissions were still occurring (DHSS 1985).

The 1980s witnessed a considerable increase in the number and activities of advocacy and campaign groups relating to people with mental health needs and people with learning disabilities. This was in part due to the emphasis on consumerism and the need to listen to clients. The need for client involvement and power in decision making was reflected in the new legislation pertaining to education, mental health and children introduced in the 1980s. The statementing process gave parents an increased legal right to participate in decisions about meeting their child's special educational needs. For the first time parents now completed a report on their hopes and expectations for their child's education which had to be taken into account when education authorities were making decisions about school provision. This legislation also stressed the need to pursue inclusive educational settings and the use of mainstream schools for people with special educational needs.

A major gap in the arguments for the widespread development of community care was the absence of solid evidence that the new system would be better for clients and their families and was capable of widespread application.

The recommendations of the Jay Report (with their associated considerable expense) were not acted upon and instead the care in the community initiative was launched in 1983 following two years of consultation. This initiative sought to provide the necessary evidence for the advantages of community based care.

In 1983 the All Wales Mental Handicap strategy was launched to run for 10 years. This was an innovative approach to provide services across Wales within a coordinated multi-agency framework incorporating health, social services, education, and housing agencies (Ayer 1997). The strategy was supported by central government and Welsh Office commitment to special funding arrangements. Evaluations reported similar findings to the demonstration projects; in particular, advances had been achieved in individual planning, increasing residential and day care provision and developing a family centred approach to services. This provided evidence of the ability to implement a community based approach when substantial additional funding and a clear commitment to development was present. However, limitations and slower-than-expected progress were also observed (Beyer et al 1991, De Paiva & Lowe 1992).

The wider view – a different perspective

Some evidence of good practice was reported in services for people with mental illness and people with learning disabilities. This included innovative projects in respite care, community nursing, family placement schemes for children, group homes, landlady schemes and sheltered accommodation projects. Common across most good practice projects were: people committed to local change; a focus on action; locally integrated services; focus on local neighbourhoods; and a cohesive multidisciplinary team approach, often involving partnerships between statutory and voluntary agencies (Audit Commission 1986).

Unfortunately the good practice was overshadowed by limited widespread progress. Despite being 15 years into the targets set in 1971 (DHSS 1971) progress fell below what would have been anticipated. Hospital beds for people with learning disabilities had reduced by only 39% (some long term admissions were continuing), community residential places had increased by 56%, and a 52% increase in day care facilities was reported.

Services for people with mental illness showed similar slow progress after 1975: a 45% reduction in hospital beds; 41% increase in residential accommodation; and 17% and 16% increases in day hospital and day care provision respectively. It was noted that increasing numbers of people with mental illness were using hostels for the homeless and coming to the attention of the police and prison service. The scale of people 'slipping through the net' of community care was graphically illustrated in a study of media reports into people with mental illness being reported in local and national newspapers during 1988 (Weleminsky 1989).

Health and social services authorities were accused of 'putting the cart before the horse' and putting people at risk by failing to develop adequate community services prior to reducing hospital provision due in part to an 'obsessive concentration' on closing hospitals (DHSS 1985). A series of other major criticisms were made of the current state of care in the community that reflected very badly on the government of the day (see Box 10.4).

Further to the information presented in these reports, evidence was mounting to show the institutionalisation of some community based services. Clients were reported to have limited choice, be living in large units in institutional living accommodation, were spending long periods of time unoccupied, and there was limited attention to individual needs (Barr & Fay 1993, Cambridge & Hayes 1994, Donnelly et al 1994, Sinson 1993). Ironically, in some localities many people appeared to be leaving hospitals only to live in community units that were bigger and just as remote (see also Box 10.5).

The evaluation of community care for people with mental illness and people with learning disabilities in Northern Ireland reported that the majority of people discharged from hospital preferred their new environments (Donnelly et al 1994). It provided limited evidence of increased

---

Box 10.4 Additional deficits in community care implementation (DHSS 1985, Audit Commission 1986)

- Fragmentation and confusion over roles and responsibilities of services (including housing, social security, voluntary agencies)
- Decreasing and fragmenting system of accountability for public funds
- Failure to transfer adequate funds from hospitals to community based services
- New grant allocated funds penalising statutory services when building new community facilities
- Rate capping restricting the ability of local authorities to raise finance
- Perverse incentives through payments from social security funds to assist people to enter residential accommodation, but not available for home based support such as home help
- Difficulties in obtaining adequate numbers of qualified staff
- Increasing public disquiet about the limited support provided to people discharged from hospital
- Difficulties in obtaining emergency admissions and 'out of hours' support
- Failure to support the 90% of people with mental illness, 85–90% of people with learning disabilities, and their families who had always lived in the community and never been admitted to hospital

---

Box 10.5 Indicators of deterioration in services at 5 year evaluation (Cambridge & Hayes 1994)

- Increasing number of 'homes' in which the exterior and interior appearance is institutional
- Growing gaps in accountability as services moved away from public provision
- New types of purchaser/provider monopolies are excluding clients
- Increased fragmentation and wasteful duplication in services
- Emphasis on 'contract culture' resulting in increased 'short termism', instability and confrontation
- Two tier system emerging as a result of care management

---

self-help skills and greater life satisfaction for some clients. However, for the majority of clients it reported no significant skills development 2 years after discharge and only limited integration into community settings. Further evidence of institutionalisation of the structure, location and running of community based facilities was found.

Flexible services

It became apparent during the mid 1980s that not all people residing in hospitals could easily be integrated into community based services. In particular, among people with mental illness, special attention would have to be given to those with acute mental illness, the elderly and those who had been in hospital for many years. Among people with learning disabilities, those with additional sensory impairments, those with challenging behaviour, people with multiple handicaps, and people with learning disabilities who also had a mental illness would require more specialist services. The Short Report (DHSS 1985) and the Audit Commission (1986) both supported the continuing efforts to develop effective community based care, and argued that additional funding was necessary. Together both reports made over 150 recommendations (many of which remain relevant) for improving community care spanning services offered by health, social services, general practitioners, housing associations, police, transport services, multidisciplinary teams and researchers.

Activities

Read through the recommendations outlined in the Short Report/Audit Commission.

- List those that are within your sphere of responsibility.
- Outline any action you can take as an individual or a team member that could contribute in bringing about the relevant recommendations within your service.

The continued emergence of community care

The late 1980s witnessed a re-think as to how community care should proceed (see Chapter 7). To date, the 1990s have seen a fragmented and inconsistent approach to community based services. In the early and mid 1990s this was characterised by defensive and 'crisis response' policies from a government coming under

increasing pressure and the impending prospect of defeat at a general election. Policies have tended to focus on short term problems and lacked long term vision and commitment.

It is difficult to be clear about the exact nature of emerging services from the start of the 1990s to date; however, it is possible to identify four emerging themes and chart their development. These aspects of services are: the need to hear the client's / carer's voice, the focus on individualised packages of care, the development and variation in localised services, and the continuing questions about the feasibility of community care (see Chapter 7).

Activities

- Compile a list of voluntary and private service providers in your locality.
- Contact two services and obtain any written information about the services they provide.
- Keep information in a resource file, along with the information obtained by fellow students.
- Compile a list of the advantages and disadvantages of utilising a mixed economy of care approach in relation to the services required by two clients you are working with.
- Try to arrange a visit to facilities that interest you if you are unfamiliar with them.

REPRESENTATION

The growth of self- and supported advocacy groups (and challenges to the independence of 'professional advocacy') in the 1980s increased the voice of the clients (Conlan & Day 1994, Gates 1994). This was matched by the increased pressure exerted by campaign groups at local and national levels. Many campaign groups increased their political lobbying skills and the development of coalitions between groups kept community care very clearly a political issue. People with mental illness and people with learning disabilities have become increasingly visible on local committees, service planning forums, interview panels, in teaching students on professional training courses, as well as presenting papers at local and national conferences.

However, the complexities of preparing people to make decisions, and at the same time getting professionals to relinquish power, continue to require much more work (Braye & Preston-Shoot 1995).

The implementation of the care management approach (SSI 1991a, SSI 1991b) in April 1993 highlighted the importance of access to independent representation for clients and carers when negotiating packages of care. This is further emphasised in the Carers (Recognition and Services) Act 1995, which was implemented in England and Wales in April 1996. This for the first time provides carers who provide 'regular and substantive' care with a legal right to have an assessment of their abilities and needs undertaken, separate from the assessment of the person being cared for. This legislation is in some ways limited by its vagueness in defining 'regular and substantive care' and allowing this to be defined locally with the variation this will bring. There are no current plans to extend this Act to Northern Ireland, although the principles of it will be applied as good practice and represented in trust guidance to staff. However, carers do not have a legal right to assessment and therefore could be less empowered than their counterparts in England and Wales. Potentially this could be a very valuable piece of legislation but it is too early to confirm the degree of commitment to it in practice. Similarly the future contribution of the Disability Discrimination Act 1995 towards equality of treatment in society and improved representation of people who are disabled remains to be seen (see Chapter 9), particularly in the light of the fact that the government introduced this legislation after preventing the passing of a much more comprehensive bill on disability discrimination (see Cooper & Vernon 1996 for a further examination of government tactics).

Three major limitations of progress on representation to date exist. Firstly, the limited availability of accessible information means that many people remained disempowered through lack of knowledge about their rights, acceptable standards, available services and opportunities for redress (MHF 1996). Secondly, attention tends to focus on more able and vocal people with mental illness and people with learning disabilities. Those with more profound disabilities or long term debilitating mental illness continue to be largely under-represented. Finally, outdated restrictions and the bureaucratic requirements of the criminal justice system (such as the need of all witnesses to be open to cross-examination in a court room) and because of the desire by the Crown Prosecution Service in England and Wales (or the corresponding bodies in other UK countries) to have a good chance to win every case (Williams 1995). Such rigidity mitigates against charges being brought against people accused of serious crimes against people with learning disabilities and people with mental illness and seriously restricts any claims about equality of treatment or a real commitment to hear their voice.

Activities

- Outline the opportunities available for the clients of service in which you work to have their voice heard.
- In discussion with the clients, identify the factors that assist and those that impede their views being expressed.
- Outline an incident when you disagreed with a client, and provide an explanation of the way in which you attempted to ensure the client had an adequate opportunity to express his views.
- Reflect on how you feel when clients and their carers disagree with you. What influence do you think these feelings may have on your response?

LOCAL INITIATIVES

Initially, it was an option for health authorities to take NHS Trust status. The option was removed in 1993 and it was made a compulsory change. All statutory health services are now organised through NHS Trusts (Health and Social Services Trusts in Northern Ireland due to integrated departmental structure). It was believed that the new structures would provide more opportunities to develop services that are sensitive to demographic, cultural and ethnic characteristics of local communities.

Trusts are provided with devolved budgets and increased autonomy to make decisions about local service priorities and developments. Considerable variation exists in relation to how mental health and learning disability services have been incorporated into new trusts. Only a few trusts exist that provide solely learning disability or mental health services. Many previous mental health and learning disability specialist structures have either been combined into a joint mental health/learning disability trust, or incorporated into either community or acute hospital trusts.

Some evidence for innovative approaches to care exists in the increasing range of specialist services that are now available within community settings. Up until the late 1980s specialist services were largely located within hospital settings and involved a person residing in hospital. With the development of increased outpatient clinics and the deployment of specialist therapists into community settings, the need for hospital admission for specialist treatment has reduced. Specialists working in community settings include those with additional professionally recorded qualifications (primarily from nursing backgrounds) working within specific services, for example cognitive behaviour therapists, child and adolescence therapists and behavioural therapists (learning disability).

Further to this, individual practitioners have been undertaking specialist training at differing professional and academic levels in such areas as working with people with autism, complementary therapies, family therapy, counselling, and working with people who have been abused (physically, sexually or emotionally) or who have perpetrated abuse. These are emerging and often over-subscribed services with long waiting lists. Their contribution to comprehensive community based services and the increased quality of life of people who use the services is yet to be assessed.

The future of remaining hospitals is to be 'centres of excellence' providing specialist treatment for people who cannot effectively be treated in community settings. Within services for people with mental illness, specialist treatment is likely to focus on people who are acutely ill and those who need a secure environment. In services for people with learning disabilities both these facilities will exist, along with facilities for people with challenging behaviour and possibly people with multiple and complex learning and physical disabilities (Mansell 1993).

Market forces have had an influence on the development of specialist services. The presence of specialist services can be a valuable advertising tool and lead to significant income by 'selling' services to local areas who do not wish to set up their own services. This in turn has led once again to the centralisation of some services which invariably reduces choice for clients and carers and can lead to difficulties in maintaining contact and integration if the services are not local. The development of specialist services for professionals other than doctors has contributed further to the reduction of adherence to medical models of treatment and, to some extent, the reduction of medical supremacy in mental health and learning disability services.

Health promotion is now a key aspect of all health professionals working within services. The importance of mental health promotion for all people was noted in the *Health of the Nation* (DoH 1992). More recently, guidelines have been issued to assist services reach targets set for the reduction of mental illness and, in particular, suicide. A separate strategy document has also been issued to highlight the need for health promotion among people with learning disabilities and how these may need to be adapted to respond to the specific needs of clients (DoH 1995).

THE FEASIBILITY OF COMMUNITY CARE

Criticism of community care and increased public concern over the quality of services (in particular support for people discharged from hospital) continued in the 1990s. The new devolved structure of more autonomy to trusts also enabled the government to deflect criticism of community care policies towards the poor implementation of their guidance by local trusts.

Inquiries were undertaken into individual

situations such as the care of Christopher Clunis (Ritchie 1994), a man with a violent psychiatric history who killed someone, and service-wide issues such as the quality and range of services available (Audit Commission 1994, Emerson & Hatton 1994, MHF 1996). These raised yet further evidence of local and central problems identified in the 1980s, such as unclear roles and responsibilities, inconsistent approaches to care and treatment, a reluctance to take unpopular decisions, the unavailability of emergency support for families, fragmented, uncoordinated multidisciplinary working and the growth in institutionalisation in community based facilities.

Failings in mental health legislation, in particular being unable to make people continue treatment after discharge from hospital, were identified. In response to the criticisms, a 10 point plan for mental health services was outlined in 1993 (Box 10.6). The Mental Health Task Force was also set up in 1993 to assist with the implementation of community care policies. This introduced the plans for the establishment of

---

Box 10.6 Ten point action plan for mental health services (Burns 1994)

- Increase power to supervise people discharged from hospital by introducing 'supervised discharges' and increasing to 1 year period of time that people can be recalled to hospital
- Publish DoH review of 1983 Mental Health Act
- Publish a revised code of practice for the Mental Health Act, with specific attention to the criteria for compulsory admission
- Review guidance in relation to people discharged from hospital to reduce number of inappropriate discharges and increase coordination of support
- Increased level of training for key workers in mental health services
- Development of enhanced information systems relating to people with mental illness and the development of supervision registers
- A review of the standards of care for people with schizophrenia in hospital and community settings
- Mental Health Task Force to develop work to assist movement towards locally based care
- GP fundholders and health authority purchasing plans to cover the essential needs of the mental health service
- Specific attention to developing best practice in London services to be taken forward by the London Implementation Group

---

supervision registers and the new power of supervised discharge. Supervision registers were introduced in 1994, and the Mental Health (Patients in the Community) Act was implemented on 1 April 1996, under which Community Treatment Orders can require a discharged person to reside in a specific place, and attend for medical treatment and rehabilitation.

Challenges have also been directed at the conceptual basis of community care as well as the progress of implementation. The origins of community care have been challenged as 'a crisis management strategy of the 1950s' (Goodwin 1990) and 'built out of economic necessity rather than any clinical utility' (Baldwin 1993). Community care has also been challenged as being based on a series of false assumptions, including the assumptions that: there is a community; the community cares; formal structures can be separate from communities; and communities are safe and friendly places (Skidmore 1994). The assumption that it is possible to separate treatment (to be provided by the state) and care (to be provided by the community) has also been challenged (Goodwin 1990). Calls have been made to replace the model of community care with more local, neighbourhood, people centred approaches (Baldwin 1993) and to replace normalisation with 'inclusion', which stresses citizenship and acceptance of people for what they are (DHSS NI 1995).

Conclusion

It has been consistently noted in this chapter, from research on a small and large scale, that progress has been uneven. The past decade has clearly seen an increased emphasis on the economics of community care and how money may be saved, despite recurrent calls for additional funding. Few, if any, new person centred service principles have emerged. Indeed it appears that no new vision of services has been presented since the early 1970s.

There is mounting evidence of microinstitutionalisation, growing size of community 'homes', and the re-emergence of viewing people in need of care as a burden. This has recently been noted in the reluctance of GPs to admit people with learning disabilities to their register, due in part to fears that their treatment would be expensive (Singh 1997). It could also be argued that the growth in prevention of learning disabilities by genetic counselling, prenatal testing only if the parents are agreeable to an abortion, failure to treat people with learning disabilities as comprehensively as others, and the re-emergence of Eugenic attitudes is related to the rising materialism of the 1980s and 1990s.

No matter how you view the evidence, the case for community care as a means to improve the quality of life for all people with mental illness and people with learning disabilities remains unproven. A proper assessment will involve a shift in research methodology away from quantitative approaches which often look only at superficial issues (Baldwin 1993). A deeper and more sustained investigation of the effects of community care on the life of people and their families, as they view it, is required.

Any research of this kind undertaken should give specific attention to people who have always lived in the community, since there has been comparatively little investigation into their abilities and needs and those of their families.

Professionals and all other 'stakeholders' need to be open to seriously questioning the services they offer against the benefits to people who use the services. The conclusion of the Short Report (DHSS 1985) continues to provide a key criterion against which progress should be measured when it concludes that 'in the final analysis, the outcome will be judged next century, neither by the location of care, not by the nature of the agency providing care, nor even by the category of staff concerned, but by the quality of care available and the extent to which individual needs are catered for'.

 Activities

Compile a list of evidence that community based services in your locality are effective:

- Highlight any gaps of difficulties in the services available.
- Compare your list your with group members and, where possible, with some clients of the service.
- Identify the areas of similarity between you and the clients you talked with. Reflect on why differences (if any) exist and how their presence may influence your ability to effectively evaluate services from a client's perspective.

REFERENCES

Atkinson D, Jackson M, Walmsley J 1997 Forgotten lives: exploring the history of learning disabilities. British Institute of Learning Disabilities, Kidderminster

Audit Commission 1986 Making a reality of community care. HMSO, London

Audit Commission 1994 Finding a place: a review of mental health services for adults. HMSO, London

Ayer S 1997 Services for people with learning disabilities in the UK. In: Gates B, Beacock C (eds) Dimensions of learning disabilities. Baillière Tindall, London, pp. 265–295

Baldwin S 1993 The myth of community care: an alternative neighbourhood model of care. Chapman and Hall, London

Barr O 1995 Normalisation: what it means in practice. British Journal of Nursing 4(2):90–94

Barr O 1996 Developing services for people with learning disabilities which actively involve family members. A review of recent literature. Health and Social Care in the Community 4(2):35–43

Barr O, Fay M 1993 Community homes; institutions in waiting?. Nursing Standard 7(41):34–37

Barton R 1959 Institutional neurosis. J. Wright, Bristol

Barton R 1976 Institutional neurosis, 3rd edn. Wright, Bristol

Beyer S, Todd S, Felce D 1991 The implementation of the All Wales Mental Handicap strategy. Mental Handicap Research 4(2):115–140

Braye S, Preston-Shoot M 1995 Empowering practice in social care. Open University Press, Buckingham

Brown H, Smith H 1992 Normalisation: a reader for the 1990s. Routledge, London

Burns T 1994 Mrs Bottomley's ten point action plan. Psychiatric Bulletin 18:129–130

Burton M 1997 Intellectual disabilities: developing a definition. Journal of Learning Disabilities for Nursing, Health and Social Care 1(1):37–43

Cambridge P, Hayes L 1994 Care in the community: 5 years on. Life in the community for people with learning disabilities. Arena, Aldershot

Conlan E, Day T 1994 Advocacy – a code of practice. Mental Health Task Force User Group/HMSO, London

Cooper J, Vernon S 1996 Disability and the law. Jessica Kingsley, London

De Paiva S, Lowe K 1992 Service contacts: change over five years in a total population sample. Mental Handicap Research 5(1):33–48

Department of Health 1992 Health of the nation. HMSO, London

Department of Health 1993 Services for people with learning disabilities and challenging behaviour of mental health needs: a report of the project group. (Mansell Report) HMSO, London

Department of Health 1995 Health of the nation: a strategy for people with learning disabilities. HMSO, London

Department of Health and Social Security 1969 Report of the committee of inquiry into allegations of ill treatment of patients and other irregularities at Ely Hospital. HMSO, London

Department of Health and Social Security 1971 Better services for the mentally handicapped. HMSO, London

Department of Health and Social Security 1972 Report of the Committee of Inquiry in Whittington Hospital. Cmnd 4861. HMSO, London

Department of Health and Social Security 1974 Report of the Committee of Inquiry into South Ockenden Hospital. HMSO, London

Department of Health and Social Security 1975 Better services for the mentally ill. HMSO, London

Department of Health and Social Security 1976 Fit for the future. The report of the committee on child health services. (Court Report) HMSO, London

Department of Health and Social Security 1979 Report of the committee of inquiry into mental handicap nursing and care. (Jay Report) HMSO, London

Department of Health and Social Security 1979 Report of the Committee of Inquiry into Normansfield Hospital. Cmnd 7357. HMSO, London

Department of Health and Social Security 1985 Community care, with special reference to adult mentally ill and mentally handicapped people. (Short Report) Second Report from the Social Services Select Committee. HMSO, London

Department of Health and Social Security Northern Ireland 1995 Review of policy for people with a learning disability. DHSS, Belfast

Donnelly M, McGilloway S, Mays N, Perry S, Knapp M et al 1994 Opening new doors: an evaluation of community care for people discharged from psychiatric and mental handicap hospitals. HMSO, Belfast

Emerson E, Hatton C 1994 Moving out: impact of relocation from hospital to community on the quality of life of people with learning disabilities. HMSO, London

Gates B 1994 Advocacy: a nurse's guide. Scutari, London

Gilbert T 1993 Learning disability nursing: from normalisation to materialism – towards a new paradigm. Journal of Advanced Nursing 18(5):1604–1609

Gladden R 1997 Legislation and social policy over the past 100 years. In: Gates B (ed) Learning disabilities, 3rd edn, pp. 311–319. Churchill Livingstone, Edinburgh

Goffman I 1961 Asylums: essay on the social situation of mental patients and other inmates. Penguin, Harmondsworth

Goodwin S 1990 Community care and the future of mental health service provision. Avebury, Aldershot

Hall V, Russell O 1985 Community mental handicap teams: the birth, growth and development of the idea. In: Sines D, Bicknell J (eds) Caring for mentally handicapped people in the community. Harper & Row, London, pp. 38–47

Mansell J L 1993 Services for people with learning disabilities and challenging behaviour or mental health needs. HMSO, London

McCarthy M 1989 New politics of welfare: an agenda for the 1990s. Macmillan, Basingstoke

Mental Health Foundation 1996 Building expectations. Opportunities and services for people with a learning disability. Mental Health Foundation, London

National Development Group 1977 Mentally handicapped children: a plan for action. HMSO, London

National Development Team 1978 Helping mentally handicapped people in hospital. London, HMSO

Neugebauer R 1996 Mental handicap in medieval and modern England. Criteria, measurement and care. In: Wright D, Digby A (eds) From idiocy to mental deficiency. Historical perspectives on people with learning disabilities. Routledge, London pp. 20–43

O'Brien J 1992 Developing high quality services for people with developmental disabilities. In: Bradley V J, Bersani H A (eds) Quality assurance for individuals with developmental disabilities. Paul Brookes, Baltimore, pp. 7–35

Race D 1995 Historical development of services. In: Malin N (ed) Services for people with learning disabilities. Routledge, London, pp. 46–78

Ritchie J 1994 The report of the committee of inquiry into the care and treatment of Christopher Clunis. HMSO, London

Rogers A, Pilgrim D 1996 Mental health policy in Britain. A critical introduction. Macmillan, London

Rose S 1993 Social policy: a perspective on service developments and interagency working. In: Brigden P, Todd M (eds) Concepts in community care for people with learning difficulties. Macmillan Educational, London, pp. 5–29

Singh P 1997 Prescription for change. Mencap, London

Skidmore D 1994 The ideology of community care. Chapman and Hall, London

Sinson J 1993 Group homes and community integration of developmentally disabled people: micro-institutional-isation. Jessica Kingsley, London

Social Services Inspectorate 1991a Assessment and care management. A practitioner's guide. HMSO, London

Social Services Inspectorate 1991b Assessment and care management. A manager's guide. HMSO, London

Tyne A, O' Brien J 1981 The principles of normalisation. Campaign for Mental Handicap, London

Weleminsky J 1989 Slipping through the net. National Schizophrenia Fellowship, Surbiton

Williams C 1995 Invisible victims. Crimes and abuse against people with learning difficulties. Kingsley, London

Wolfensberger W 1989 Reflections on a lifetime in human services and mental retardation. Mental Retardation, 29(1):1–15

Wolfensberger W, Thomas S 1994 Obstacles in professional human services culture to the implementation of social role valorization and community integration of clients. Care in Place 1(1):53–56

Wright D, Digby A (eds) 1996 From idiocy to mental deficiency. Historical perspectives on people with learning disabilities. Routledge, London

Children

Julie S. Taylor   Owen Barr

At the end of this chapter the student will be able to:

- **appreciate the gradual evolution of separate policies for children**
- **describe how deprivation underpins many social difficulties encountered by children**
- **discuss socioeconomic factors that are associated with child policy issues**
- **discuss some future trends for child care services**
- **summarise some of the research that informs future trends in policy**

Introduction

The provision of separate legislation and public policies for children is essentially a 19th-century phenomenon. In previous centuries children were broadly categorised in two ways. First, in terms of meeting their developmental needs, they were classed as dependants along with the old, the crippled and the mentally ill. Second, in terms of accountability to the rest of society they were simply classed as 'appendages of' or belonging to a family and therefore the responsibility of their father or legal guardian. It is possible to trace a degree of evolution in children services before this time but they are generally within the confines of the family unit. These changes include the responsibility for ensuring their protection, education and welfare. Until the 19th century it was more or less sacrosanct that child care was not the work of government intervention and not therefore a sphere of public or social policy.

Before industrialisation, the economy of Britain was largely agrarian based and supported by local cottage industry. The ethos of self-sufficiency and autonomy that underlined the rural lifestyle effectively reinforced the culture of family boundaries against public or state intervention. The effect of industrialisation during the 19th century was therefore an impetus towards the revision of policies towards children. Living conditions in the cities for families migrating from the countryside were harsh and children were especially affected by the squalor and disease. The novels of 19th-century writers such as Charles Dickens portrayed the social effects of poverty, illiteracy and poor hygiene on the well-being and development of children. However, because these living conditions were occurring in cities they could not remain hidden, despite the existence of utilitarian policies such as the Poor Law Amendment Act.

Increasing public exposure of the circumstances of children through philanthropists, pressure groups and concerned individuals led to the beginnings of reform and eventually a series of policies that recognised the essential needs of children. New working practices were introduced that outlawed the use of child labour and new health care measures were gradually introduced. In the early part of the 19th century, the provision of health care for children was more or less the same as for the remainder of society, in that it was marked by inaccessibility. However, by the middle of the century, the beginnings of a health visitor service were beginning to appear and in major cities such as London, Liverpool and Manchester children's hospitals were built.

By the end of the 19th century an up-turn in the economic performance of Britain, along with the changes in social policies towards children, created a social environment that would still be be broadly familiar today. Bilton (1987) referred to this as 'the march of time'. A clear delineation developed between home and work, with work becoming a separate and external activity. The slight rise in individual wealth allowed mothers to stay at home with their children, assuming the role of housewife and mother, while fathers became the breadwinner. However, by far the most important gain in public policies for children was in the area of education.

Activities

- Read one of Charles Dickens's classics (e.g. *David Copperfield* or *Oliver Twist*) to try and get a feel of what life was like for children during the 19th century.
- Organise a seminar with your colleagues to discuss your findings.

EDUCATION

Earlier education acts had made education compulsory, along with the provision of proper school building. However, during the 19th century attitudes to teaching and the function of school became more complex. Traditional ideas mixed with new unconventional strategies. Some held on to the belief that school was only about training and preparation for a life of work. It should therefore be rigorous and disciplined and promote concepts such as respect and obedience. Others took their views from enlightened philosophers such as Rousseau. They argued that childhood was a fragile period of life and therefore education should be a mechanism for cushioning children against the tough world of adulthood that lay ahead (Bell & Harper 1977). This latter view was supported by emerging work in the field of psychology. Sigmund Freud, the Austrian psychiatrist, argued that childhood traumas frequently predetermined the attitudes and behaviours of adult society (Aries 1960, Bell 1977, Mitchell 1989).

During the early years of the 20th century, schools began to improve because it was recognized that education was an investment in terms of having a more competent workforce in the future. The Liberal government, supported by Labour MPs, was able to introduce new policies that had a direct link with health care. These included the provision of school meals in primary schools and a local levy to provide free school meals for the less well off. Local authorities were also empowered to carry out medical inspection of school children. In time this created links between local health and education authorities that led to a system of school clinics in every area (Jones 1991).

Major reforms in education also formed a large component of the new welfare state that was introduced after the Second World War as part of the Beveridge plan to eliminate the 'five giants' (want, ignorance, idleness, squalor and disease). The Butler Act, named after R A Butler, the Conservative minister who guided it through parliament, was a cornerstone in government policy towards the care and support provided by government for children. Effectively the Act led to a raising of the school leaving age and, as a result, a substantial school building plan. Post primary education was divided into three categories: grammar schools for the more intellectually minded; technical colleges for those who wished to pursue industrial or apprenticeship type careers; and secondary modern schools for the remainder of children. Most controversial of all was the introduction of an 11-plus test that was used as a guide for the separation of children (Jones 1991).

POVERTY

Despite changing definitions of poverty and subsequent arguments as to whether it should be described as relative or absolute, the last few years have shown that too many children are brought up in deprived circumstances. Recent estimates suggest that as many as one child in three in Britain grows up in circumstances of poverty (National Commission of Inquiry into the Prevention of Child Abuse 1996), and more British children are considered to live in poverty than in any other EU country (Kenny 1997). This is an appalling indictment and recalls Alexis de Tocqueville's 1835 *Memoir on Pauperism*, where it is clear that our dependency culture certainly goes back to the Elizabethan poor laws. He states that 'among very civilised people, the lack of a multitude of things causes poverty; in the

savage state, poverty consists only in not finding something to eat' (Smith et al 1997). In examining the differences in health in 678 electoral wards of the northern region of England, it was found that death rates were four times as high in the poorest 10% of the population than in the richest 10% (Phillimore et al 1994). It is ironic that in spite of the plethora of social policies that exist to protect children, there still remain such anomalies, especially in a country that prides itself on being civilised.

DEPRIVATION

A useful summary of the current divisions in equity or fair distribution of services are provided by Bebbington & Miles (1989). This comparative study related the likelihood of children being admitted to care. The results of this study provide a graphic illustration of one particular effect of social deprivation. The evidence from this study concluded that the rate of children admitted into care from poor districts is higher than would have been anticipated from family relationship predictors alone. It is clear, therefore, that children from poorer backgrounds have a far greater likelihood of being taken into care than those who enjoy no overcrowding, or who come from a white background in a household where there is a reasonable income and two carers are present (see Table 11.1). Bebbington & Miles conclude that deprivation

Table 11.1 Two children compared*	
Child A	Child B
Aged between 5 and 9	Aged between 5 and 9
No dependence on social security benefit	Head of household receives income support
Two parent family	Single adult household
Three or fewer children	Four or more children
White	Mixed ethnic origin
Owner occupied house	Privately rented accommodation
More rooms than people	One or more persons per room

*The chances of being taken into care of Child A are 1 in 700; those of Child B are 1 in 10 (Bebbington & Miles 1989).

is the single most important factor among all children who require statutory support and that 'coming from a poor ward has an independent effect on the probability of entry' (p. 357).

Activity

Using a broad definition of health, offer four reasons why it would help our overall health policies if we could provide effective support mechanisms for children.

TACKLING INEQUALITIES

It has been calculated that the lives of more than 2000 children a year could be saved if the overall mortality rates for the total population were aligned with those living in the top two social classes (Reading 1997). Bradshaw (1993), quoting the Breadline Britain Survey, showed that about 2.5 million children go without at least one of the things they need every day (e.g. 3 meals a day, toys, or separate bedrooms for boys and girls at age 10 plus). Alongside this, the same report showed that the number of people claiming benefit has doubled in 10 years. Reading (1997) argues that community nurses trying to help children in poverty are ineffective if the government does not concurrently implement effective strategies to reduce the presence of inequalities. Health care professionals need to consider how clearly ill-health and deprivation are linked; in so doing they can contribute some key strategies for future action. Lessons can possibly be learned from an examination of international conditions.

Bradshaw (1993) offers the following explanations as to why so many of our children are suffering deprivation:

- economic: there is high unemployment coupled with an increased labour supply and less labour demand, lower wages and more long term unemployment
- demographic: increases in marital breakdown and births out of wedlock contribute to a deprived population

Box 11.1 Pictures of deprivation

- 1 in 3 children grow up in poverty
- Britain has more children living in poverty than any other EU country
- 2.5 million children go without at least one of the things they need every day
- infant mortality is five times higher in class V than it is in class I
- 85% of parents claim income support at some stage of their lives
- there are 150 000 recognised homeless people in Britain, many of whom are single parents with families
- 100 000 children in England and Wales have school attendance problems
- Britain has more single parent households than anywhere else in Europe
- £11 billion per annum is spent on housing benefit

- 85% of parents claim income support at some stage of their lives
- indirect tax: the rises in VAT, National Insurance and poll tax all have a negative effect, particularly so because benefits have not risen in line with earnings. As well as this, household rents continue to rise, thus increasing the rate of homelessness.

INTERNATIONAL PERSPECTIVE

There are lessons that can be learned from other countries that enjoy better morbidity and mortality rates. Wilkinson (1996) questions why it is that the life expectancy of children is better in countries where income differences are small. Bangladeshi children are one of the most materially deprived groups in society yet children from this country are the least likely to die in their first year of life (Graham 1993). It has been argued that neither medical care nor genetics can explain why it is that one country should be healthier than another, as it does not appear to correlate with individual risk factors (for example smoking or diet). Life expectancy is higher in Greece, Iceland and Italy than in the USA and Germany, even though the former are not as economically powerful. Greece, Iceland and Italy, among others, all seem to enjoy a better social fabric which in turn leads to better overall health (crime rates, suicides and so forth) and is not related to national wealth. Wilkinson (1996) suggests that simple economics are not the reason why other countries are more successful in creating more satisfying living conditions within which families can bring up children safely and in a stimulating way. Relevant factors include:

- a strong community life
- more public space, which in turn means more social space
- they are less antisocially aggressive
- they are more caring. (Wilkinson 1996)

Wilkinson (1996) puts forward the unusual idea that Britain was at its healthiest during the inter-war period. Aside from the obvious existence of high levels of poverty, poor housing, sanitation and education, Wilkinson contends that Britain was a more egalitarian society and the quality of life for residents in particularly difficult areas was better than other epidemiological indicators would suggest.

 Activity

Find out about the life expectancy of the countries mentioned above and discuss any other reasons why there should be this difference. What lessons are there here for health care workers?

PARTICIPATIVE/INCLUSIVE POLICIES

Programmes provided by various social and health care agencies tend to target the socially disadvantaged, even though definitions of 'at risk' groups can be tenuous at best. Whilst there are probably positive effects to this policy, the methodological flaws in their accurate identification restrict effective analytical evaluation (Gough 1993). Researchers prefer to advocate community strategies because they have the beneficial effect of avoiding traps such as focusing on minority pockets of the population. Tuck (1995) sums it up well, when maintaining

that there are three strands that link these problems: social deprivation leads to socioeconomically impoverished neighbourhoods where it becomes difficult to provide a safe and healthy environment. Material, social, interpersonal and intrapersonal barriers in families and social deprivation can all prevent people from achieving the parenting standards to which they aspire. And, in interaction with other factors, social deprivation then leads to increased psychosocial stress which may lead parents to physically injure or neglect their children.

All of these factors are interrelated. There is therefore a need for population based strategies that are inclusive to address them. Drawing from Garbarino's work, Tuck suggests that it is not just neighbourliness that counts, but also the degree of social support available, which needs to be sufficient to offset the dangers of disadvantage. Belsky (1984) offers a convincing explanation as to why some people are better able to cope with adversity than others. He describes this as a balance of stress on the one hand, with coping capacity and support on the other.

TARGETING SERVICES

Any measure of health status should be based on a concept of health and this should ideally be a very broad model (Bowling 1995). The underlying philosophy of most definitions remains that of the World Health Organization (1978), that is that health is a state of complete physical, mental and social well-being and not merely the absence of disease or infirmity. Generally there have been moves away from a disease model towards an understanding of health that encompasses quality of life (Bowling 1995). Even so, 'well-being and happiness are extremely vague concepts, open to marked attitudinal bias' (Rutter et al 1995, p. 1) and consequently many descriptions of health still tend to employ disease specific terminology.

The Health Survey for England 1995 confirms that nine out of ten children are in 'good' or 'very good' health (Department of Health 1997b). Recent advances in paediatric practice and medical technology have resulted in a fall in neonatal mortality rates, although it must be pointed out that many of those 'saved' by technologies such as ECMO suffer significant neurological disability as result of their treatment (Pearn 1997). It becomes clear, though, that it is complicated to separate physical health from social and psychological well-being.

Children suffering from chronic illnesses have an increased risk of secondary symptoms of psychosocial illness (Nolan et al 1986) and as psychological diseases are so often linked (e.g. depression and suicide), it makes sense to look at psychosocial disease as an integrated whole (Rutter & Smith 1995). Goodman (1997) suggests that children with conduct difficulties (and by implication their parents) are not a health problem, but one for social and educational services. In support of this, White (1997) cites studies that show that 20% of children are maladjusted or distressed and dismisses most of them as ordinary misery rather than pathology. Whatever your view of this opinion, abdicating responsibility does not change the fact that the welfare needs of these groups still exist and strategies for dealing with this need to be made by someone. Brushing problems under the well-worn carpet is neither historically nor domestically sound practice.

In terms of policy, the medical evidence linking poverty and ill-health was ignored by the Conservatives until 1995, when the Minister of Health announced a £2.4 million research programme on this issue (Kenny 1997). According to Kenny: 'The real problem with the Conservatives' approach is that it puts too much emphasis on lifestyles and behaviour and ignores the social and environmental causes of ill-health' (Kenny 1997, p. 13). Britain spends 23% of its gross domestic product on welfare and, in relation to other industrial countries, this is quite small (Numas 1997).

As we have seen, statistics still show higher morbidity and mortality in the lower socioeconomic groups and some of this may be linked to the environment. For example, damp housing can lead to respiratory problems and there may be nutritional difficulties because of reduced income (Spencer 1993). Social dependency is associated with low birth weights, probably because of the effects on maternal nutrition (Habicht et al 1974), although Brooke et al (1989) claim that smoking rather than social factors is the most important determinant of birth weight. The Third National Cohort Study (Golding et al 1986) predictably found huge social class differences in health in the first 5 years of life. Headaches, wheezing, bronchitis, mouth breathing and repeated accidents were much more prevalent amongst the lower social classes, but they conclude that this is because of behaviour rather than morbidity. Maternal smoking, the number of children in the household and the type of neighbourhood are all contributory factors. This seems to place the blame on the parents again, although another explanation is provided by Graham (1986). She concurs that although the lower social classes smoke more, this is seen as a necessity rather than a luxury and has pay-offs as a coping strategy.

Mortality figures, however, do not indicate healthiness, and morbidity data is much harder to obtain (Power & Fox 1991), but studies on failure to thrive (FTT) and non-intentional injury support this view. Equally, there is an observable association between low SES and symptoms of asthma (Demissie 1995). Dubowitz (1991) further argues that other measures of ill-health, such as iron deficiency anaemia and dental disease, are also likely to be significantly higher in this population. Certainly this is confirmed in Scotland, where tooth decay is accepted as a disease associated with social deprivation (Jones et al 1997). Other diseases are showing similar trends. A 3 year study in North Thames region shows that overcrowding and lower social class are associated with an increased risk of meningococcal and pneumococcal meningitis (Rees Jones et al 1997).

 Activity

List the strengths and weaknesses of such communitywide compensatory approaches and discuss the impact they could have on your clinical work.

LIVING CONDITIONS

There is evidence that the neighbourhood wherein one lives makes a significant contribution in regard to the effects of deprivation on individuals (Garbarino 1986). Blackburn (1991) describes Townsend's concept of 'environmental poverty' as a lack of, or lack of access to, essential amenities, where account should also be taken of noise, dirt and pollution. In this context it is clear that poor community provision makes good and positive child care all the more difficult. Melton et al (1994) investigated the social processes that were related to increased incidences of child maltreatment. This study produced evidence of a direct correlation between an increasing incidence of reported child abuse in specific geographical areas and deteriorating social conditions in terms of unemployment, drug and alcohol abuse and other forms of antisocial behaviour.

Revised policies are clearly needed, especially in the areas of unemployment, housing and education. However, the government seems to consider that these social issues are the responsibility of the individual and not the state. The dominant values in health education/promotion remain elitist and individualist (Rodmell et al 1986). Inherent behind much of our current policy and welfare provision is the notion of participation (Hill & Bramley 1986), for example the poor should be able to fend for themselves. It has been pointed out, however, that although disadvantaged families may have the same values as those who are materially better off, their coping mechanisms can be compromised and they are sometimes unable to avoid potentially harmful behaviours (Baldwin et al 1993).

CHILD ABUSE

Child abuse is 'anything which individuals or institutions do, or fail to do, that directly or indirectly harms a child or damages the prospects of safe and healthy development into adulthood' (National Commission of Inquiry into the Prevention of Child Abuse 1996, p. 2).

Abuse is multidimensional in that there are physical, emotional and sexual aspects contained within it; however, each dimension is inter-related (Cleaver et al 1995). From this perspective it is clear that many children are currently being brought up in less than optimal circumstances, the consequences of which to their well-being can only be measured in the longer term. From this definition it is estimated that about 1 million children are harmed in Britain every year. It is paradoxical that at present there are only about 32 000 children who are considered to be at risk and placed on the child protection register and the number of new cases that are added has gradually fallen in recent years (Department of Health 1996). This figure, when broken down, reveals that 40% are believed to be at risk of physical injury, 33% are neglect cases, and 22% are thought to be at risk of sexual abuse.

FAMILY SUPPORT

Blackburn (1991) refers to 'cultures of poverty' and 'cycles of deprivation' which are based on the assumption that parents bring the values and behaviours from their own upbringing to the care they give their children. Even if external forces maintain these things, the family is seen to be responsible. This is reinforced by the media – child criminals are typically portrayed as 'little monsters', and their parents rather than society are generally held responsible. However, as Blackburn maintains, although there may be significant differences in their practices, if we look at their approaches (beliefs and attitudes) we find mostly similarities. Low income families are forced to make sacrifices and compromises that better off families do not even have to consider, often because they have no choice (Blackburn 1991).

Finerman (1995) criticises the many studies that direct attention at parents (especially mothers as the main caregivers) for not complying with health regimes. She suggests that over the years these have become more accusatory, with parents being blamed for a perceived failure to provide adequate care. Based on her research in Ecuador and Guatemala, she reveals that many parents who in fact fit models of parental neglect and incompetence are actually proactive health seekers who are forced to make inequitable decisions about the allocation of scarce resources. The Walker Rivers study within a deprived inner city area clearly showed that despite the vulnerability of children in such areas, parental irresponsibility was belied by the high levels of commitment shown by parents in the community (Wallace 1992). Even in families that had become involved in the child protection process, despite high levels of stress most parents showed a strong commitment to their children (Thoburn et al 1995).

CHILDREN'S RIGHTS

It has been argued that childhood is a period of dependency, powerlessness and subservience. As a result, in certain circumstances, children have become a target for oppression in terms of abuse or neglect. The creation of a bill of rights for children has been interpreted as a way of addressing this anomaly at a national and international level. In line with this idea, the United Nations adopted the Convention on the Rights of the Child that became a legally binding agreement between the twenty nations that ratified it. This agreement is applicable to all children, irrespective of class, ethnicity, religion or family background. Signatories were expected to develop policies that would facilitate a full expression of the child's view in any decision making. They were also required to ensure that children were given a high priority in terms of allocating economic resources and the provision of specific facilities. It was from this agreement that legislation such as the Children Act emanated.

The Children Act 1989

The Children Act 1989 for the first time articulated the rights of the child and the child's parents. It laid down principles (Box 11.2) to underpin the future care of all children, including children with disabilities (incorporating learning disabilities and mental health). These principles reflect the principles within the UN Convention on the Rights of the Child, ratified by the UK government in 1991. Central to services for children was the need to ascertain the views of children and their parents through a comprehensive assessment. This assessment should take a longer term perspective for children with disabilities and may lead to a corresponding longer term package of care.

Common themes of multidisciplinary teamwork, the right to challenge professional decisions, and the need for increased accessible information are incorporated into the new vision of children's services. Hospital and community trusts are also required to maintain a register of children with disabilities in their locality to assist with local and flexible service development. Facilities providing residential care for children were also brought into the registration and inspection arrangements for all community residential facilities.

Box 11.2 Principles underlying current children's legislation and services

- The child has rights.
- The welfare of the child is paramount and the state and parents have a duty to safeguard and promote the welfare of children. Intervention should be open to challenge.
- Whenever possible, children should be brought up and cared for within their own families.
- Services are provided in partnership with parents and carers.
- Staff should work with and support families, and parents with children in need should be helped to bring up their children.
- The views of the child, parents and carer are taken into account.
- Children should be kept informed about what happens to them and should participate when decisions are made about their future.
- The welfare of the child must be the paramount consideration when a court makes a decision about the upbringing of a child.
- Parents should continue to have parental responsibility. They should be kept informed and participate in decisions, even when their children are no longer living with them.
- Any delay in proceedings is likely to prejudice the child's welfare.
- A court should only make an order if it would be better for the child than making no order at all.
- All decisions must be based on the checklist of considerations as outlined in the legislation.

INTERAGENCY SUPPORT

The ability to provide a healthy environment is strongly related to an individual's ability to cope with the balance between stress, coping capacities and social support. Perceptions of one's own ability to deal with adversity is also an important influence, and neighbourhoods can be targeted as being in need of social support before they reach a stage where problems become difficult to alleviate (Chamberlin 1988). Tuck (1995) provides what is referred to as a cognitive-social constructionist model as an attempt to account for the links between social dependence, psychosocial stress and harm to children, illustrating the processes that characterise these. Although there is no agreed definition of psychosocial stress, 'parenting in social disadvantage has an extraordinary potential to be perceived and felt by those who experience it as extremely stressful' (Tuck 1995, p. 128). Tuck goes on to suggest that parents facing disadvantage have to make painful, if not impossible, choices regarding their children's needs in order for the family to survive – for example, the choice between the child's overall safety and the child's need to play outside. The relative lack of protective influences for such people makes it more difficult for parents to reduce the stresses associated with child rearing.

Good standards of material and emotional care are strongly related to the quality of housing. Recognising this and providing interagency support has been incorporated into some government strategies, for example the Children Act: 'On registration of a child, the initial plan should include a comprehensive assessment. Its purpose is to acquire a full understanding of the child and family situation in order to provide a sound basis for decisions about future actions' (Home Office et al 1991, p. 31).

An important question that needs to be addressed is why some people are influenced by difficult circumstances and others are not? It has been suggested that the key differentiation lies in the presence of mediating responses or moderating factors that occur within family units and that may facilitate individual adapta-

tion and permit normal childhood development (Elder et al 1986). Some compensatory programmes that have been introduced in certain areas are based on this premise and they contain many indicators for policy makers.

Low parental tolerance for stress can be modified by the spouse; poor ability to manage acute crises and child provocation behaviours can be buffered by educational programmes and increased coping resources, and compensatory factors can be used to limit aggression within families, for instance through community support. Alloway & Bebbington (1987) also underlines the importance of social support in mediating the effects of stress and preventing adverse physical and mental reactions to it. The National Committee for Prevention of Child Abuse (1983) provided support for first time mothers, offering videos, pamphlets, education classes and visits by aides. In another similar scheme, the US Head Start programme assumed that the environment was the key determinant of intellectual and social development, but after 15 years of compensatory family support they had to conclude that this was not the antidote to poverty (Zigler et al 1978).

Likewise, a controlled study examining the effectiveness of social support to parents of handicapped children found few differences in outcome when compared to the control group (Glendinning 1986). Gibbons et al (1990) reviewed compensatory programmes and found that although the studies were small and experimental design was not used, consistently positive results were reported. Further, they looked at four major studies in the USA (compensatory programmes with the abused) which they concluded to have disappointing and inconsistent research results.

 Activity

An example of a programme that advocates a 'transitional model' that permits the development of buffering methods to reduce the 'inter-generational transfer of the cycle of disadvantage' is provided by Wolfe (1987). Order this publication from your school library and set up a seminar to consider the beneficial effects of such a programme for specific client group.

Conclusion

There are differences between morbidity and mortality and we need to look more widely in examining this. It is all too easy for health care professionals to suffer from the insidious and pervasive *Struthio camelus* syndrome, ostrich symptoms that manifest themselves in the inherent belief that even health policy, never mind a wider social policy, is not our remit. However, the NHS is not the only body that will make a difference to the lowering of mortality rates (Griffiths 1991). So, although the previous government extolled the virtues of the market place and patient power, they made little provision for the needs of children.

The NHS has become characterised by less privacy and less information for patients, despite the *Patients' Charter* (Griffiths 1991). Recent concerns regarding the numbers of registered sick children's nurses are still disturbing. Only 50% of health authorities purchase community children's nurse services, and only 1 child in ten can get a 24-hour children's nurse service (Department of Health 1997a). These health inequalities have been reinforced both directly and indirectly by policy decisions and strategies. As Hill & Bramley (1986) illustrate, this occurs in the following ways:

- there are inequalities in the geographical distribution of health services
- these services are underused by deprived groups
- there are differences in service provision to deprived groups (for example the length of GP consultations).

However, there are hopes for the future. The new government has asked the Chief Medical Officer, Sir Donald Acheson, to update the Black Report. The Labour government is ideologically more sympathetic to the recommendations of the Black Report, but it is at the same time committed to low public spending (Kenny 1997) and it will be interesting to see their response to the CMO's task (see Box 11.3).

If we look forward with optimism, we may note that the Prime Minister Tony Blair does

---

Box 11.3 Deprivation

- deprivation lies at the heart of social injustice
- the root causes of many social problems arise within a context of deprivation
- increased mortality is associated with deprivation
- although harder to measure, higher morbidity is associated with deprivation
- most of these 'problems' are not a personal responsibility
- those who succumb to the adversities arising from deprivation are relatively few
- there appear to be mediating factors that work protectively with some individuals
- social policists should explore these 'buffers' in developing future strategy

---

seem to recognise that legitimate reasons may exist as to why single parents do not work and has proposed using national lottery money to fund after-school clubs to give such parents time to work (Prescott 1997). He has also talked about a 'workless class'. This underclass costs the country £11 billion a year in housing benefit alone and although it is proposed that greater incentives to work will be introduced, the prevailing view still seems to be one of workshy scroungers. One thing that distinguishes those living in disadvantage is the lack of choice open to them – some proposed policy decisions may reinforce this and perhaps the indirect effects will be felt by health care professionals.

Activities

- Order from your school library a copy of Graham G 1990 *Contemporary social philosophy*. Blackwell, Oxford. Critically review Chapter 7, 'Children in society', and then discuss the responsibilities of families and society towards children.

- Have a 'Mad Hatter's Tea Party'. On a small piece of card each write down one thing that you believe is more a personal, rather than a policy, responsibility regarding child care. Place these cards in a hat and take it in turns to pull one out. On your turn, read the statement on the card out loud and then give three good reasons why this is not a personal responsibility. Then open it to discussion with the rest of the group.

REFERENCES

Alloway R, Bebbington P 1987 Buffer theory of social support. Psychological Medicine 17:91–108

Aries P 1960 Centuries of childhood. Cape, London

Baldwin N, Carruthers L 1993 Henley Safe Children Project. Interim report. NSPCC/University of Warwick, London

Bebbington A, Miles J 1989 The background of children who enter local authority care. British Journal of Social Work 19(5):349–369

Bell R, Harper V 1977 Child effects on adults. Embaum, New Jersey

Belsky J 1984 Child maltreatment: an ecological integration. American Psychological Journal 35:320–335

Blackburn C 1991 Poverty and health: working with families. Open University Press, Milton Keynes

Bowling A 1995 Measuring disease. Open University Press, Buckingham

Bradshaw J 1993 Social disadvantage and child health – an overview. In: Waterston T Perspectives in social disadvantage and child health, pp. 3–8. Intercept Ltd, Newcastle-upon-Tyne

Brooke O G et al 1989 Effects on birth weight of smoking, alcohol, caffeine, socioeconomic factors, and psychosocial stress. British Medical Journal 298:795–801

Chamberlin R W 1988 Beyond individual risk assessment: community wide approaches to promoting the health and development of families and children. Maternal and Child Health Clearing House, Washington D C

Cleaver H, Freeman P 1995 Parent perspectives in cases of suspected child abuse. HMSO, London

Demissie K 1995 Social class gradient in childhood asthma: the nature of the link and issues of measurement. Health Sciences Public Health. Mcgill University, Canada

Department of Health 1996 Children and young people on child protection registers year ending March 31 1996, England. HMSO, London

Department of Health 1997a Health services for children and young people in the community: home and school. HMSO, London

Department of Health 1997b The Health Survey for England 1995. HMSO, London

Dubowitz H 1991 The impact of child maltreatment on health. In: Starr R, Wolfe D A The effects of child abuse and neglect. Issues and research, pp. 278–294. Guildford Press, New York

Elder G H, Caspi A, van Nguyen T 1986 Resourceful and vulnerable children: family influences in hard times. In: Silbereisen R K, Eyferth K, Rudinger G Development as action in context, pp. 167–186. Springer, New York

Finerman R 1995 'Parental incompetence' and 'selective neglect': blaming the victim in child survival. Social Science Medicine 40:5–13

Garbarino J 1986 Where does social support fit into optimising human development and preventing dysfunction? British Journal of Social Work 16 (Supplement):23–27

Gibbons J, Thorpe S, Wilkinson P 1990 Family support and prevention: studies in local areas. National Institute for Social Work/HMSO, London

Glendinning C 1986 A single door: social work with the families of disabled children. Allen and Unwin, London

Golding J, Butler N R 1986 Birth to five. Pergamon Press, Oxford

Goodman R 1997 Child mental health: who is responsible? British Medical Journal 314:813–814

Gough D 1993 Child abuse interventions. A review of the research literature. HMSO, London

Graham H 1986 Caring for the family. Health Education Council, London

Graham H 1993 Hardship and health in women's lives. Harvester Wheatsheaf, New York

Grice A, Smith D 1997 Blair launches crusade for welfare reform. The Sunday Times: 1, 4th May

Griffiths D 1991 Politics of health. Pulse Publications, Fenwick, Ayrshire

Habicht J P, Lechtig A, Yarbrough C, Klein R E 1974 Maternal nutrition, birthweight and infant mortality. In: Elliott K, Knight J Size at birth, pp. 353–370. Elsevier, Amsterdam

Ham C 1992 Health policy in Britain. Macmillan, Basingstoke

Hill M, Bramley G 1986 Analysing social policy. Blackwell, Oxford

Home Office, Department of Health, Department of Education and Science, Welsh Office 1991 Working together under the Children Act 1989. HMSO, London

Jones C M, Woods K, Taylor G O 1997 Social deprivation and tooth decay in Scottish schoolchildren. Health Bulletin 55(1):11–15

Jones K 1991 The making of social policy in Britain, 1830–1990. Athlone Press, London

Kenny C 1997 Milk of human kindness is back in fashion. Nursing Times 93(25):12–13

Melton G B, Flood M F 1994 Research policy and child maltreatment: developing the scientific foundation for effective protection of children. Child Abuse and Neglect 18 (Supplement 1)

Mitchell F 1989 Unpublished essays. University of Ulster

National Commission of Inquiry into the Prevention of Child Abuse 1996 Childhood matters. Volume 1: The Report. Stationery Office, London

National Committee for Prevention of Child Abuse 1983 Perinatal positive parenting. Final report, collaborative research of community and minority group action to prevent child abuse and neglect. National Committee for Prevention of Child Abuse, Chicago

Nolan T, Pless I B 1986 Emotional correlates and consequences of birth defects. Journal of Pediatrics 109:201–216

Numas R 1997 New Labour, new NHS. Nursing Times 93(20):30–31

Pearn J 1997 Paediatrics I: infancy and early childhood. British Medical Journal 314:801–805

Phillimore P, Beattie A, Townsend P 1994 The widening gap. Inequality of health in northern England, 1981–1991. British Medical Journal 308:1125–1128

Power C, Fox J 1991 Health and class: the early years. Chapman and Hall, London

Prescott M 1997 Labour assault on single mothers. The Sunday Times 1, 1st June

Reading R 1997 Poverty and the health of children and

adolescents. Archives of Disease in Childhood 76(5):463–467

Rees Jones I, Urwin G, Feldman R A, Banatvala N 1997 Social deprivation and bacterial meningitis in North East Thames region: three year study using small area statistics. British Medical Journal 314:794–795

Rodmell S, Watt A 1986 Conventional health education: problems and possibilities. In: Rodmell S, Watt A The politics of health education. Routledge and Kegan Paul, London

Rutter M, Smith D 1995 Psychosocial disorders in young people, Introduction, pp. 1–7. Wiley, Chichester

Smith D, Woods R 1997 How will they fare? The Sunday Times, 14 May London: 5.6

Spencer N 1993 Social disadvantage and child health – a medical perspective. In: Waterston T Perspectives in social disadvantage and child health, pp. 9–15. Intercept Ltd, Newcastle-upon-Tyne

Thoburn J, Lewis A, Shemmings D 1995 Paternalism or partnership? Family involvement in the child protection process. HMSO, London

Tuck V 1995 Links between social deprivation and harm to children. A study of parenting in social disadvantage. Unpublished PhD thesis. Social Sciences, Psychology. University of Warwick, Coventry

Wallace B 1992 Studying life in the inner-city – can research benefit the people who live there? Health Education Journal 51:144–148

White S 1997 Commentary: ordinary misery should not be mistaken for pathology. British Medical Journal 314:816–817

Wilkinson R G 1996 Unhealthy societies. Routledge, London

Wolfe D A 1987 Child abuse: implications for child development and psychopathology. Sage, Newbury Park

World Health Organization 1978 Constitution. In Basic Documents. WHO, Geneva

Zigler E, Valentine J 1978 Project Head Start: a legacy of the war on poverty. Free Press, New York

3

Wider issues

This section will discuss current and future trends in health and social care provision from a national and international perspective. The chapters will also consider the effects of demographic trends and the changing nature of ill health and social care in terms of the funding and administration of health and social care services. In conclusion, the final chapter will provide the student with views on the way ahead or future directions for health and social care.

International health care provision

Simon Smith

After studying this chapter the student will be able to:

- **describe the philosophical ideas behind health policy in a selection of countries**
- **discuss the political influences that shape health policy within a country**
- **outline the approach to health policy in a selection of post-industrial nations**
- **explore an approach to health care in the People's Republic of China**
- **discuss variances between countries in the delivery of health care**

Introduction

This chapter will address health care provision with an international perspective and focus on the major philosophical/moral ideologies which drive different health care systems and social policy.

Commonalties and variances within alternative delivery systems will be identified in the role of government, organisational structure, the role of health care professionals, and resource allocation. Case study examples will focus on the USA, Germany, Sweden and China.

Comparisons are difficult to make across international boundaries and the aim is not to undertake in-depth analysis of that. The aim will be to increase the reader's understanding of different approaches toward health care provision and the philosophical and moral issues driving these alternative systems.

ISSUES IN HEALTH CARE

The ethical issues facing all nations are broadly similar, that is;

- concern with equity
- concern about access to care
- distribution of care
- cost containment
- quality of care.

In evaluating other health care systems it is useful to consider how they attempt to deal with these issues. A general trend within post-industrialised nations in the post-war period has seen an enormous growth in the role of the state in the provision of health care. You will have read in preceding chapters that until this time health had tended to be the responsibility of the medical profession, charitable institutions and local government. There had been an evolutionary process of greater state involvement, with such notable changes as the enforcing of minimal sanitary conditions and running of public health programmes to financing the overall provision of medical care.

In order to function, advanced capitalist societies required a healthy population – the means of production. It was essential therefore to have some means of health care provision for the population at large. As economies thrived and developed during this period, greater affluence enabled a greater proportion of disposable income to be spent on health care. This greater wealth and expenditure also helped to finance and support the rapid development and sophistication of medical care and treatments.

In this period, then, efforts were made in an attempt to ensure equitable and equal access to this sophisticated technology. The aim was to remove the principal barrier that would have limited access in the past, that of ability to pay. Different countries approached this with a mixture of publicly and privately funded services. There was a proliferation in the growth and modernisation of hospitals, where much of the new technology would be centred.

The direction of policy has undergone a radical rethink through the 1980s and 1990s, as has the political thinking behind the provision of health care. The dream of eradicating ill-health has gone and new approaches to providing health care and managing the 'unwieldy monster' that became the health services had to be found. There have been a number of reasons for this reassessment:

- concerns about the spiralling costs of health care
- concerns over justice and equitable distribution of health care
- radical reassessment of the goals of health policy
- the influence of a New Right political philosophy.

Concerns about the spiralling costs of health care

There were many reasons that led to concerns about the rising costs of health care. Increasing specialisation in medicine led to developments in treatment and new technology. While offering benefits, these developments had a high financial cost in the research, development and eventual service provision. The infrastructure to support this, including the emergence and growth of many other groups of professional and support workers, had major cost and organisational implications.

As new treatments were discovered, a demand was created for them. This raised increasing ethical concerns – if we can treat or cure a particular medical ailment, is it right or just to deny it to any member of society. Over the course of the 20th century we have moved through the era of hope and expectation that we could meet all health care demand. Now we have entered an era of rationing, that is we will do what we can afford. There remain serious moral concerns for health policy decision makers in ensuring an even and fair distribution of health care resources.

Justice and equitable distribution of resources

Despite the increase in resources directed toward health care, there remains the perennial problem of inequitable access and variation in quality. Throughout all the advanced Western industrialised nations the percentage of gross domestic product dedicated toward health care has steadily increased. The poor or lower social classes, however, still suffer a greater proportion of ill-health and proportionally have benefited less from the 'improved' health services. Even in the most advanced health systems, distribution of care can be uneven with the 'best' concentrated in centres of excellence which attract the best doctors and the most advanced technology. There can be arguments to support this in relation to the sophisticated treatments that can be offered and the improved outcomes that result. On the other hand, a consequence may be that more isolated rural areas may suffer as a result through a shortage of even the most basic of health services.

Radical reassessment of the goals of health policy

There was a realisation that perhaps the focus of health policy must be redirected in order to achieve better outcomes. There was a growing recognition that it was necessary to treat the cause of ill-health rather than focusing on the effect. This effectively meant that rather than chipping at the 'tip of the iceberg' one had to go under the surface. The problem was more complex and embraced areas other than health such as welfare, housing and social ills in society.

There was a school of thought that felt that state provision stripped people of a sense of responsibility for their own lives. Individual responsibility for health and welfare began to dominate many of the ideas on health and welfare. All of the industrialised nations have grappled with this problem of providing a reasonable standard of health care for their citizens while at the same time trying to contain the escalating costs of an unwieldy system. This chapter will look at a selection of these countries to try to compare and contrast the efforts made and lessons to be learned. All of the countries have a mixture of private and state health care provision. There can be wide variation on

the amount of gross domestic product spent on health care (Abel-Smith 1994).

Activities

- What factors have contributed to higher costs in the United Kingdom?
- What evidence is there for the problem of inequitable access in the United Kingdom?

THE US EXPERIENCE

In keeping with being one of the world's richest countries, the United States of America spends more per capita than any other country on health care (OECD 1992). Some commentators say this is not surprising as per capita health expenditure rises relative to per capita income and the USA experiences the highest per capita income. In looking at the US experience it is worth giving consideration to the issue of whether money can buy better health care for a country's citizens. In evaluating the health system one would have to consider: concerns with equity; equal access to care; equality in distribution of care; issues of cost containment; and the quality of care provided.

In the USA health care is provided by a mixture of state and private provision. The involvement of government in health care provision on a large scale dates back only to the mid 1960s. This was following the introduction of two federally based programmes, Medicaid and Medicare, which were a response to the apparent failure of the market based model of health care in the USA (Brannigan 1995).

Medicare

Medicare is a federally supported insurance plan for those over 65 with permanent disabilities or end-stage renal disease. It comes in two parts: one which covers the need for hospital care and the other which covers the cost of physician and non-hospital services. It is an entitlement plan which is subsidised through taxation. Areas not covered under Medicare include long-term institutional care, drug prescriptions, and eye and dental care.

Medicaid

In contrast to Medicare, Medicaid is a joint state and federal-based system aimed at covering the health needs of the poor and disadvantaged. Funding under this scheme attempts to fill in the gaps left out by other means of provision. However, it is not an entitlement plan and there is no guarantee of eligibility under this scheme. While the federal government provides guidelines and a proportion of the cost, individual states administer the programme and set their own eligibility guidelines. As state Medicaid expenditure has risen, states have countered this by limiting eligibility and benefit entitlement under the scheme. Not surprisingly, provision varies between states with many setting a qualification bar well below the federal poverty level with the result that many people have no medical cover at all.

Other state provision

State provision also exists indirectly through tax incentives for those in employment. Those in middle to high income employment are eligible through tax-free employer paid premiums. There is also some provision made for indigent war veterans through the Veterans Administration, which provides through its own hospitals free care for those eligible.

There remain two major concerns facing the USA in relation to health policy at the current time. They are the escalating costs overall of health care and, in addition to this, the numbers of people without any medical cover at all. There remains a group, estimated at between 30 and 40 million people, who have no cover or links with the health system. If they do require care it is limited to public hospitals that are subsidised by the state and local government. Most of them receive rather inadequate medical care and when they do it is often in the latter stages of their illness, which further complicates matters.

Therefore the evidence would indicate that, despite the high overall expenditure on health care, there is wide variation in the health care experience of US citizens. In other words, there is unequal access to care, with one system for the 'haves' and another for the 'have-nots'. In terms of overall quality of care, if one considers some of the crude indicators of a nation's standard of health, then the USA performs badly. For example, judging by infant mortality rates and life expectancy, per capita expenditures of almost twice the average of OECD countries have not resulted in better health care. The only countries with worse infant mortality rates than the USA in 1987 were Greece and Turkey. Male life expectancy at birth is also closer to the bottom of the league.

 Activity

In what ways does the United States health care system differ from the National Health Service?

Rising costs in the US health care system

It is worth exploring this issue of the amount of money spent on health care in the USA and asking why it has not achieved a better outcome. Since the 1960s, the amount of money spent on health care has increased massively for a combination of reasons. Between 1950 and 1980, medicine increased its share of the gross national product from 3.5% to 9.1%. Rublee (1992) suggests four reasons for this:

- health care inflation tends to exceed that of the national economy
- increased uptake of services by patients
- increase in age and size of population
- increasingly costly treatments becoming available.

As in most Western industrialised nations, the early years witnessed a huge growth in number, size and sophistication of hospitals.

The introduction of Medicaid and Medicare in the 1960s was a response to the growing concern about inequity in the provision of care. There was less concern with cost at this time but more emphasis on meeting the health needs of the poor and the elderly. This greatly expanded the access to and, as a consequence, the demand for health care. However, there was no slow down in the growth or sophistication of hospital services. In addition, the development of neighbourhood and community health care developed in parallel with it. It increased the income for hospitals who were paid their fee – whatever it was – plus 2% (Feldstein 1992). Over this period employment based insurance schemes increased greatly. Companies were able to negotiate better rates for cover in purchasing such insurance than an individual applicant would. Such schemes became part of the employment package. One reason for this suggested by Feldstein (1992) was that health insurance is not considered taxable income. Therefore, dollar for dollar, additional income was worth more to an employee as extra health insurance than if he received a higher income on which he would pay tax. This was compounded by the high inflation in the 1970s which pushed more and more employees into higher marginal tax brackets. The result was that employee health insurance became more and more comprehensive and individuals became less and less concerned with the actual cost of health care. The most rapid increase in amount of GDP devoted to health care was between 1980 and 1990, when it rose from 9.2% to 12.1%. It is predicted that this will rise to 17% by the year 2000 (Sonnefield et al 1991) and with a rapidly ageing population could reach 37% by the year 2030. There are now concerns that the high cost of health insurance is becoming an economic burden on some companies. It is estimated by the Chrysler Corporation that health care costs added $700 to the cost of every vehicle produced compared to $246 in Japan and $223 in Canada (Hackler 1995).

An analysis of expenditure by the Organization for Economic Cooperation and Development (OECD 1992) concluded that higher US expenditure on health was a reflection of higher prices to a large extent, rather than higher volumes of health care. The purchase of health care is not limited by the usual market restraint of a direct payment at time of consumption. This is the same in all Western industrialised economies and is an attempt to ensure access to the service. Even in the USA, which is mostly privately funded, the marginal cost is covered either through taxes or through insurance premiums. However, most systems have some form of co-payments, for example prescription charges, dental and optician fees. The US system features high co-payments relative to other countries, which should act as a restraint in the demand for services. However, this has not risen much in the past 20 years relative to overall costs and as it generally accounts for only a fraction of the initial expenditure, is an even smaller fraction of the true cost for the most intensive users of the health care system (Manning et al 1987). Hence, given the lack of any disincentive, patients have a tendency to over-consume health care. In any case many individuals have insurance cover for these marginal costs, meaning there is never any direct payments at the time of consumption.

US insurance based system

There is a belief that the very existence of an insurance backed system for health care acts as a force to drive costs up. There is the incentive to over-consume on the part of the patient. Physicians are in the position where they know their patients can afford even the most expensive of procedures and the full range of diagnostic measures, so there is no incentive to limit supply. With the USA being an increasingly litigious society, it is also in doctors' interests to cover every eventuality in the event of being sued for malpractice. In addition, physicians in the USA operate on a fee-for-service payment schedule and the evidence suggests that such a system will tend to increase the overall expenditure on health care. Physicians who practice in clinics that have a lot of technology available have a tendency towards over-zealous use of it. For example those who own CAT scanners would tend to prescribe more scans, even in cases where the potential benefit to the patient is minimal. There is also the fact that as individuals have received much more comprehensive cover under employer based schemes, they feel they have 'earned' the best standard of care. Therefore physicians are responding to demand.

Moral hazard and adverse selection

Moral hazard is where insurance cover acts as a stimulus to change the behaviour of the insured and thus increases the risk. An example of this is the consumption of more health services than genuinely required or by taking little action to prevent ill-health, both of which increase the risk to the insurer. Therefore insurance with the existence of moral hazard is inclined to lead to overly risky behaviour. If insurers were able to distinguish illnesses that would have occurred even in the absence of cover, a policy could be written which would cover only this and there would be no moral hazard.

In any given population there will be variation in the risk for health insurance and insurers try to reflect this in pricing policies. Health insurance is a business and insurance companies need to make a profit. Adverse selection occurs if the policies a company offers attract a disproportionate number of bad risks and thus reduce their profits. If insurers are not allowed to price policies according to risk they will 'cherry pick' to avoid high-risk cases. The unfortunate end result of this, in an insurance based system, is that the highest premiums are charged to those who need the most care and this conflicts with the goal of equal access to care. Therefore if an individual is unfortunate enough to suffer from a chronic medical condition, he represents a 'bad' risk and may find it increasingly difficult to get adequate medical cover.

Administration costs in an insurance based health system

There are higher administration costs in an insurance based system of care. Taken on its own, the administration of Medicaid and Medi-

care is comparable with other OECD countries. The insurance overheads comprise the normal costs of providing insurance in a competitive market. These include marketing costs, accessing risk liability for insurance and verifying and processing claims. Woolhander & Himmelstein (1991) estimated that the administrative costs of insurance represented 10–13% of personal health care expenditure. In addition to this there are also administration overheads inherent in the very cost and expenditure controls, such as patient payments and utilisation review measures, introduced to curtail consumption.

Access to health care in the US system

The issue of physical access to health services in the USA is not in itself a problem. The more pertinent question is whether people have access in respect of 'can they afford health care'. The introduction of Medicaid and Medicare has to a large extent dealt with the worst of the problem of access. For those under 65 and in employment, the majority are covered through employer based insurance schemes. There remains a substantial pool, however, of about 15% of the population without any form of medical cover, representing about 35 million people. These are made up largely of those working in small firms, part-time workers and the unemployed. Those without insurance do not necessarily go without medical care but it is generally inferior, often through the emergency room, usually late in the course of an illness and as a consequence more expensive and complicated to treat.

Americans who can afford it receive technologically the most advanced medical care in the world. The likelihood is that such a system is unsustainable, that there will have to be some slow down in the form of employers, insurers and governments paring back on the comprehensiveness of cover. The effect will be to further erode access to care. The measure of the success of health policy cannot be made on the basis of excellence for a few, mediocre for some and nonexistent for others. Restricting unwarranted use is difficult. Care that is free at the point of contact has created a dynamic of increased demand, increased supply, and the development of increasingly sophisticated and costly diagnostic and treatment options. Various schemes have been proposed to deal with this problem of escalating costs without further restricting access. Some of these on a state level are considering a tax based publicly funded health care system which would sharply reduce the role of private insurers. The Garamendi proposals in California recommended replacing insurance premiums with a payroll tax by contributions from workers and employers. Regional autonomous 'health insurance purchasing corporations' (HIPC) would use these revenues to purchase medical care from private sector providers for all its residents, employed or not. This would deal with the anomaly of loss of medical cover in periods of unemployment. It was also more equitable in that it related payment to means. That is those that earned more and could afford to would pay a greater percentage, thus spreading the cost.

There were also proposals to introduce regulation of price schedules, quantity constraints and enforcing global budgets on the health care providers. On a federal level the government has tried to restrain spending with a transition to 'diagnosis related group' (DRG) payments rather than cost based payments. Another state initiative that has been well publicised was the Oregon Plan, a proposal to extend Medicaid cover to more of the poor but at the same time eliminating cover altogether for some types of medical care. The process by which they prioritised the areas to be covered was through a series of public meetings held throughout the state and the public then decided. It is possible that this system may be adopted in other states (Brannigan 1995). It is an attempt to introduce an agreed form of rationing.

It is an indictment that a country as rich as the USA should have failed to provide comprehensive medical care for all its citizens. The introduction of regulation is at odds with political ideology and the free-market system. The Health Care Reform Act, effective from 1 January 1998, has seen the lifting of health care regulation for

the first time in 15 years and once again forces hospitals to compete in a free market. With the enactment of this law New York joins 48 other states that have enacted similar laws. It is expected that academic research will suffer as a result of this leaner system as research efforts are cost intensive without offering short term benefits in relation to health care provided (Josefson 1997).

Activities

- What were the two main concerns of health policy makers in the USA in the 1980s?
- Discuss why health care costs are so high in the USA.
- Consider whether you feel Americans get value for money in the health care they receive.

HEALTH CARE IN GERMANY

Germany, in contrast to the USA, is an example of a decentralised system with effective cost control. Cover is enabled through non-profit taking insurance organisations known as 'sickness funds'. Fees are fixed and are negotiated and paid through the medical associations. Germany has been able to fix growth in health care spending to the overall rate of growth of gross domestic product (Inglehart 1991). In regard to goals of future health care systems in Germany, Schulenburg (1992) outlines three areas:

- Any system should provide equal access to all citizens. He calls this the solidarity goal because it implies a comprehensive social health insurance plan that would cover the health care costs of all.
- Competitive pricing to ensure efficiency and the best allocation of scarce resources in medical care. To facilitate this providers should have the freedom to alter prices in response to fluctuating demands.
- There should be an element of choice, that is consumers (patients) should be able to use the hospital or physician of their choice.

The system in Germany is widely regarded as inefficient. Since the Second World War the coverage by statutory health insurance had been widened so that now about 90% of Germans are insured in the statutory scheme.

One reason that has pointed directly to inefficiencies in the German system concerns hospital care, where the average length of stay was 15.6 days in 1985. Hospital based care accounts for the biggest drain on any country's health care costs. In those countries where length of hospital stay has successfully been shortened, with consequent increased turnover of beds, it makes for a more efficient use of this costly resource. In Germany there is a higher than average number of beds, an above average rate of admissions and a longer length of stay, all of which contribute to overall health care costs. In contrast the United Kingdom is below average in all three respects and offers a much more cost-effective system.

There are a number of reasons why such a system has been slow to change. One is political. Webber (1991) suggests that as a consequence of the proportional representation electoral system, the federal government, to be re-elected, must secure the support of 50% of the electorate. As a consequence, most of the interest groups, with their varied opinions, have their concerns represented in government. These include the medical profession, trade unions, employers' organisations, the health insurance funds and so on. There are frequent coalition governments and decision making frequently ends in negotiation, compromise and maintenance of the status quo.

There are also financial reasons for long hospital stays. German hospitals are reimbursed on a per diem basis whereas in the United Kingdom hospital trusts operate within annual prospective budgets. In countries where an intense effort has been made to reduce the length of stay and increase the turnover, the time in hospital tends to be treatment intensive and consequently more costly. Where hospitals are paid per diem, more profit is made out of days that are not treatment intensive and so longer stays are in the interests of such hospitals. In short there is a motivation for early discharge in one and

for longer in-patient stay in the other. There are other factors that contribute to this inefficiency. There is a poor flow of information between office based physicians and hospitals. This is compounded by the fact that the office based physicians do not have access to the diagnostic or laboratory services in the hospital. What generally happens in Germany is that tests and diagnostic procedures that could be done as an out-patient are carried out after the patient has been admitted to the hospital, adding to the length of hospital stay. This happens even if the tests have already been carried out by the office based physicians. This lack of communication between hospital and community based services has another effect in that patients stay longer in hospital because hospital doctors are reluctant to discharge since they are unsure about the nature of care following discharge. The practice is to keep the patient in hospital until they are well recovered. This is exactly the opposite to the policy that operates within the United Kingdom.

The German Medical Association (Kassenarztliche Vereinigungen)

The office based physicians are the gatekeepers of medical care in Germany. Every patient who is covered by a statutory sickness fund must consult such a physician to access the system. They provide ambulatory care, prescribe drugs and medical appliances and decide who requires hospital care. While these physicians are private practising general practitioners, the patients do not directly pay them for a consultation. All physicians are obliged to be members of their *Kassenarztliche Vereinigungen* (KV) in order to receive remuneration for treating sickness fund patients. The level of payment is negotiated beween the sickness funds and the KV. It is worked out on a system of points for different activities consisting of about 2500 items. For example a telephone conversation rates at 80 points while a home visit has 360 points. The value in German marks of each point is variable and is used as a means of containing the rising costs of medical care. The value is derived from the sum of all points submitted by physicians in a particular region. If more services are provided than expected, the point value is less and if less than expected, then the point value increases. Cost control measures have been incorporated into this system of payment since 1983 under the Health Insurance Structural Reform Law. This is very cleverly done by linking the point value to the total number of persons insured to the average increase of wages of those insured. Thus Germany has become the first country that explicitly defines by law the percentage of income spent for medical care. Physicians receive their payment from their KV which is in turn compensated by the sickness funds. The medical association is a very powerful lobby in Germany and they have been very successful in achieving substantial salaries such that they belong to the highest income group in society. Germany is very generously supplied with doctors, with about 2.7 per 1000 population in 1986. This is expected to increase substantially over the next few years due to the numbers entering medical school. In 1970 the enrolment number was about 4500 students whereas by the mid 1980s the figure had increased to between 11 000 and 12 000 annual enrolment. Some attempts have been made to reduce this *Arzteschwemme* (physician glut) by reducing numbers entering university, by increasing the length of training and by introducing more restrictive licensing procedures for foreign physicians. This has been successful in containing costs to some extent in that while physicians' salaries remain high, they have been held in check to a point where, in real terms, they have decreased. In the early 1970s physicians earned about 6.5 times the average wage and by the late 1980s this was reduced to about 3.5 times the average wage.

Activities

- Why was the German system considered an inefficient health care system?
- Explain how Germany has managed to slow down the amount of gross domestic product spent on health care.

Reunification of Germany

In October 1990 the former socialist East Germany reunited with the Federal Republic of Germany. This was clearly going to cost a lot of money in terms of modernising the old East German infrastructure, including the national health service that existed. Most of the existing hospitals were outdated and in a state of disrepair with obsolete equipment. Per capita income in East Germany had been considerably lower than in the West. However, rather surprisingly, statistics on physician, dentist and hospital bed numbers resembled closely the figures of West Germany. Nevertheless the system was much less advanced and technologically deficient and Schulenburg (1992) suggests that much of the physician's time was spent on administration of the old national health service, which was structured on a strict hierarchy. On 1 January 1991 the West German sickness fund was extended to include all of East Germany. Not unexpectedly, there were deficits in the sickness funds and these deficits were made up by transfers from the West German fund and 'solidarity' payments made by the pharmaceutical industry. It will take some years to modernise the old structures in the East, at quite considerable expense to the German economy. These costs include the modernisation of infrastructure not directly related to health, such as transportation, telecommunications and housing costs that will run into billions of dollars. Health care reforms are presently underway. The state will continue to provide 'core services' which will be state funded and planned. However, there is discussion and debate as to what should be included in these 'core services' and over elements of health care for which there should be direct charges.

The future in the unified Germany

It is interesting to look at the German unification because it throws some light on individual motivation in relation to health care. Not only did physical and administrative changes have to take place but also individual attitudes and philosophies about the role of the state in the welfare of its citizens. Practically overnight there was a transformation from a socialist system with state control of practically every aspect of a person's life and choices to a free-market system. In relation to health care, individuals could no longer rely on the paternalism of the state for health care provision but now had to take action on their own initiative. It is very much the thing now to criticise paternalism in health care, either by health care professionals or by the state. There is a general movement for the recognition of individual rights in health care by the promotion of autonomy and the facilitating of choice. For the former East Germans this represented their whole culture being turned on its head.

Schubert-Lehnhardt (1995) explores this experience in the unified Germany. The socialist interpretation of the responsibility for health is based on the belief that all the interests of society are the same and consequently the government has the right to create norms and values for all its citizens. In East Germany, based on this philosophy, there existed large-scale medical and dental check-ups and an obligation to be vaccinated against certain diseases, all of which reinforced this view of the locus of responsibility. Schubert-Lehnhardt suggests this leads to a dissociation of individual responsibility for aspects of their health, not just through apathy but through a fostered dependence created by the state. Individual responsibility and initiative was forbidden or discouraged. Having been used to a culture where matters such as check-ups and vaccinations were organised for you, individuals now had to ask for such things. There are some concerns among physicians that some diseases that were thought to have been eradicated could recur because of this. Also school health checks detected preventable health problems at an early stage whereas now they have to be asked for, with the result that problems may be detected much later when they are more difficult and more expensive to treat.

There are certainly good aspects of the old socialist system that many feel have been lost, aspects such as social justice and collective responsibility for one's fellow man, particularly the 'weaker' members of society, and the sense of security inherent in the knowledge that the state would always be there to look after matters of health care. The autonomy and freedom of choice in a free-market is often theoretical. That is, the degree of choice is dependent on the laws of the free-market system. In essence the freedom of choice is governed by the means at the disposal of the person to pay for that choice.

There is also the question which arises in free-market systems, favoured by the New Right movement, of categorising health care as normal goods or service. In any free-market system individuals can buy goods and services as they choose. Health and medical care is difficult to categorise alongside the normal goods and services available in society. One cannot equate medical care with engaging a builder to carry out work on one's house. Historically the provision of medical services has been one of an unequal relationship between supplier and consumer. Bjorkman (1991) talks of a power relationship exercised by an active agent with specialised knowledge over a passive recipient without such knowledge or expertise. Thus in Western society the whole notion of a consumer of health care is a new concept. Bjorkman suggests this represents a novel change in recent history where governments have readily entered the domain of hitherto private relationships in order to regulate the behaviour of both sets of actors (providers and patients). In East Germany this complete change of political philosophy occurred overnight.

Activity

Discuss the differences in ideology regarding health policy between East and West Germany.

THE SWEDISH HEALTH CARE SYSTEM

Sweden's population enjoys a relatively good standard of health compared to other industrialised nations. Life expectancy is about 2 years greater than in the USA and the infant mortality rate in the USA is more than double that of Sweden (Meyer 1990). The predominant diseases facing the health system are lifestyle related, that is cardiovascular and cancers. Just as in other Western industrial nations, the proportion of elderly in the population is increasing.

Most health care in Sweden, as in the United Kingdom, is provided through the public sector. However, in the aftermath of the Second World War, Sweden, along with the other Nordic countries, developed perhaps the Western world's most comprehensive welfare system (Saltman, 1991). The modern Swedish health system began to evolve around the same time as the development of the National Health Service in the United Kingdom. This followed the publication of the Hojar Report in 1948 which set the scene for the adoption over the following years for a rather different policy tone than that of the United Kingdom (Saltman 1988). There was to be centrally based funding with locally delegated decision making, including county responsibility to develop primary health centres. The responsibilities of the county councils in health care has been expanded in recent years following reform in the early 1970s. This aimed at less central control, giving autonomy to the local councils to provide the care that was needed. They had to meet the parliamentary objective of 'Good health and health and medical care on equal terms for the entire population' (Wennstrom 1992). The fundamental principle is that all citizens are entitled to equal access to health services whatever their economic status. Hospital specialists under 1970 legislation were obligated to become fully salaried county employees. In 1970 the Primary Care Act fully endorsed and adopted a primary and preventive emphasis to future resource allocation. This preempted the adaptation of this approach in the United Kingdom by a number of years.

Administration of Swedish health services

Local decision making in Sweden is facilitated through the administration by 26 county councils which are responsible for health care delivery within their geographical boundary. They own the hospitals, which are financed by taxes raised locally. This represents 90% of the operating costs of the councils. The Swedish Health Care Act 1983 places the prime responsibility for planning of all health care on the county councils and effectively empowers them to act as independent regional health systems. They also control and regulate private health care. Unless a private practice has been given approval by the appropriate county council, any consultations with patients will not be reimbursed from social insurance. Each county has at least one central general hospital with more than 1000 beds in addition to several minor district hospitals. There are also nine regional hospitals affiliated with medical schools. They provide specialised services such as neurology, plastic surgery, radiotherapy and paediatric surgery. They serve the populations of several counties and cooperative agreements exist between the councils regarding the provision and financing of these services (Lindgren 1990).

Charges for health care in Sweden

Direct charges are nominal in Sweden for visits to the public health care facility, for prescription medicines and for visits to private practices associated with the social insurance plan. Under the social insurance plan patients do pay a fee for a visit to a doctor but only about the same price as a haircut. They are not charged any additional fees for tests, X-rays or other services. The doctors are salaried employees of the county councils. Until 1984 the county council would have received a payment for each such visit to a doctor from the central government. Following the 'Dagmar Reforms' of 1985 this fee for service payment from central funds was changed into a system of annual capitated payments channeled exclusively through the 26 regional providers. It therefore became based on the population served by the county council rather than as a fee for service. One of the reasons for this was to encourage provision of preventive and other health education and screening services as they were difficult to quantify under a fee for service system and were less likely to be provided. A central emphasis at this stage was to build up the primary care sector of the health care system, to redirect goals toward preventive measures as opposed to the curative model of care. To take account of chronic conditions, those who required frequent visits to a doctor were issued with a card that entitled them to free consultations. Also following the Dagmar reforms, salaried physicians were no longer able to give consultations in their spare time and claim remuneration under the public health insurance system. Saltman & von Otter (1990) suggest that the 1983 Health Act and the Dagmar reforms of 1985 represented the culmination of a publicly planned, regionally operated primary care based health strategy.

This health strategy had developed uninterrupted post-war until the mid-1980s, mainly because it had taken place during an extended period of Social Democratic rule. This dominant political ideology reflected concerns with distributional equity and social justice. Saltman (1991) suggests that another major influence in the health policy was the adoption by the World Health Organization during this period of an explicitly primary care based strategy. This strategy (WHO 1981) appeared to be based on the Swedish health care model.

Despite this seeming utopia in health care provision, there began to appear increasing criticism and scrutiny of the system. Like other countries the proportion of money spent on health care has been growing, although there are some signs that this has levelled off in the 1980s at about 9% of GDP. Sweden has relatively low levels of unemployment and generally experiences a high standard of living. However, there was increasing concern about the rising cost of health care. The Swedish medical system had been largely centred on hospital beds, such that 50% of all medical consultations are with doctors in hospitals. Unlike the United Kingdom, patients can make appointments with hospital out-patient departments without referral from a general practitioner. Hospital based care (in-patient and out-patient) accounts for over 70% of total health care expenditure in Sweden. Hospital care tended to generate greater costs.

Part of the reassessment was also due to changes in political thinking and part was due to economic constraints caused by economic dislocations of the world economy through the 1970s into the 1980s. There has been an increase in the influence of conservative parties at the national level and, with that, New Right economic concerns about increased productivity and reducing the public sector expenditure coming more to the fore. One aspect of this was a desire to increase the input to health care provision of the private sector. This had previously been marginal, with only about 15 000 subscribers, mainly senior executives, covered by company schemes.

There was also dissatisfaction, even among the general public, with the mainly primary care based emphasis of health care. One effect of this was that the rate of growth in specialist hospital services had been restrained. There had been movement in development of provision of surgical techniques in alleviating degenerative conditions, particularly hip replacement, cataract surgery and coronary bypass procedures. The inevitable consequence of this was increasingly longer waiting lists for such surgery. This caused dissatisfaction among Swedish citizens and campaigns for change gathered momentum, particularly in cases where treatment was life saving in nature. The familiar 'shroud waving' gave support to hospital specialists who wished to increase the funding to hospital services.

Swedish response to rising costs

The response to this in Sweden was to set up a national centre for the evaluation of medical technology to be established within the ministry. This disappointed the medical profession, which would rather have had such a body incorporated within the National Board of Health, which comprised independent professional planning and advisory bodies. In effect it was an effort to constrain over-zealous introduction of new treatments without some form of cost evaluation and consideration of the potential benefits before a demand was created. At the sharp end, or county council level, there were tentative changes to deal with the current problems. Differential payscales were experimented with, for health service staff, based on performance incentives, particularly for physicians. This broke a long term policy of wage solidarity in the public sector but it was an attempt to improve productivity and efficiency within the service. Another major shift was consideration given to contract out clinical services to the private sector. In relation to ambulatory care, there was increased use of the private sector in areas such as providing custodial care to the growing numbers of elderly. Also there were experiments in leasing out health centres to private entrepreneurs and funding private sector walk-in ambulatory clinics. Ultimately these would have been paid for by county council revenue. Elective surgical procedures were purchased by the county councils, either through two privately funded and operated hospitals or by sending patients abroad, particularly for coronary bypass surgery. In addition, private surgical groups came into existence, generally composed of publicly employed physicians working in off duty hours within their publicly funded hospitals. There were no tax incentives introduced to encourage the individual to take out private medical insurance.

In essence developments in private enterprise in the provision of health care in Sweden at this time were very much dependent on the public purse. Payment was channelled through public revenues via the county councils and professional input, for the most part, was provided by physicians already employed in the public sector. There was a feeling that it would be a short term measure to deal with the existing waiting lists and when this was dealt with it would no longer be required. Saltman (1991) draws particular attention to the absence on the one hand of support for particular privatisation activities and a New Right political ideology. As a result the response to the period of financial pressure and organisational uncertainty of the

late 1980s has been practical rather than a change in ideology in the provision of health services. There will continue to be developments in methods to meet the demand for acute hospital based care and to provide continuing social and medical care for the growing numbers of elderly, but without undermining the ideology of a principally tax-based publicly funded system. In addition there will be attempts to balance the policy formulation process between central government desires while maintaining and accommodating the system of regional autonomy in the delivery of care. In this way it is more responsive to local need.

Funding in Sweden

The health system is funded through a national insurance system providing medical, sickness and parental benefits. It is the means by which the state attempts to provide socioeconomic equality in relation to health care, but also functions as a financing instrument and an instrument of state control and supervision. There is expected to be increased demand on health care resources because of the demographic changes, principally the increase in numbers of people over 80 years of age. It is expected that in Sweden, in order to meet the increased demands, there will need to be a redistribution of resources rather than an increase in the share of GNP already allocated to health and welfare (Ham et al 1990). In terms of personnel in Sweden, with a very low unemployment rate of 1.5%, the health services are finding it particularly hard to attract staff. While medical studies remain highly attractive it remains difficult to recruit qualified physicians to some specialities and to some geographical locations. The number of physicians per 100 000 population can vary considerably from 300 in urban areas to 130 in rural areas. In addition to this there is a need to recruit staff in nursing homes, home nursing and other social services that are essential to facilitate the ongoing deinstitutionalisation of acute medical care. The net effect is that some areas have less choice and poor access to services.

Activities

- Outline the principal differences between the Swedish health care system and the British National Health Service.
- What factors led to dissatisfaction with health care among Swedish citizens?

HEALTH CARE IN THE PEOPLE'S REPUBLIC OF CHINA

It is interesting to look at the experience of the People's Republic of China (PRC) as a contrast to the experience in Western industrialised societies. There are two distinct types of medicine in modern China: Chinese traditional medicine and Western medicine. Unlike other traditional medicines, Chinese traditional medicine has a rich and theoretical base. Diagnostic methods would include observing and questioning the patient, limited physical examination, and detailed and prolonged pulse taking. Therapy involves techniques such as herbal medicines, acupuncture, moxibustion (application of heat to sites on the skin), breathing and gymnastic exercises, and flexible splinting (Sidel & Sidel 1982, p. 20). Western medical practices became more prominent in China during the early part of the 20th century. However, there is a belief that the Western model of concentrations of urban 'centres of excellence' from which well trained people and good technology would diffuse into rural areas would be ineffective in China.

In contrast to the Western experience China devotes only about 3% of gross domestic product to health care. Per capita income is more in keeping with the poorer countries in the world. China is a developing nation struggling to modernise but it has been willing to learn from the experience of the post-industrial nations. While the latter nations are now looking at issues of cost containment as health care costs spiral and benefits appear negligible, China is able to adopt health care strategies aimed at cost containment, with selective use of medical technologies. Cost containment is essential as

China so far has not experienced the rapid economic growth that provides the funds for accelerated health care spending. This perhaps in some ways is an advantage, as there are lessons to be learned from the Western experience. Also with a population of 1 billion people to serve, there are problems unique to this vast and largely rural country. In effect, problems of equality and equity encountered in any system of health care are exacerbated. It is estimated that about 850 million people live in rural areas, which increase the problem of access to health services.

Rosenthal (1992) outlined the background of the development of the health care system in China. There was a recognition of the potential, during the civil wars of the 20th century, of giving simple medical training to peasants and soldiers. The Red Army doctors also became aware of the usefulness of traditional cures and herbal medicines and, just as important, the belief and dependence of the peasants on these resources. Mao attempted to harness and modernise these traditional approaches to medicine. It was partially out of a desire to help rebuild national pride by promoting this aspect of culture but also due to scarcity of resources such as medicines, technology and doctors to administer a traditional approach to medicine.

Barefoot doctors

This is a unique system to China and was introduced by Chairman Mao in 1965 as part of the Cultural Revolution. There was a continuing problem of shortage of doctors and this was particularly so in rural areas. The system involved hundreds of thousands of rural peasants being selected and given a number of months of rudimentary medical training, following which they would be able to serve the local community, among whom they would continue to labour on a part-time basis. They would have been trained in a wide range of issues including environmental sanitation, health education, preventive medicine and primary medical care. They became known as 'barefoot doctors' because they combined this role with their agricultural work which would have been done barefoot in the rice paddies. However, the term was used simply to emphasise the fact that they remained part of the community they served and did not adopt a professional distance (Sidel 1972). Mao was said to be deeply distrustful of the medical profession, seeing it as elitist and self-serving, concentrated in the urban areas which served only 15% of the population. It created a new health provider to help deal with the continuing shortage and uneven distribution of doctors. In China attempts had been made to increase the number of medical students and to disperse them to rural areas. However, the shortage remained, as did the urban clustering of qualified doctors.

One can see this as an attempt to deal with the issues of access and distribution of health care. It could also be seen as a means of cost containment in providing a lesser qualified individual to provide health care. However, when one examines the issue of quality some people may criticise such an approach. The training and preparation of barefoot doctors varied from 3 to 6 months, with additional periods of training added on. There was a massive growth in their numbers in the early years after Chairman Mao's directive at the beginning of the Cultural Revolution in 1965. By the mid 1970s there began to appear a lot of criticism regarding the uneven training, inadequate supervision and incompetent practice of some (Sidel & Sidel 1982). There were reports of some stepping beyond the limits of their skills and expertise and treating patients in inappropriate ways. Since 1975 the numbers of barefoot doctors have declined from 1.8 million to 1.5 million in 1980, with upwards of 200 000 being dismissed as incompetent (Rosenthal 1992). Training became more complex and better controlled, with competency and theoretical exams and an expansion of continuing education.

Prevention has been of central importance since the earliest days of the People's Republic. Since the communists took control in 1949 there have been great improvements in areas such as literacy, nutrition, living standards and control of infectious diseases. Immunisation programmes

have been particularly successful considering the enormity of the task and would not have been possible without the indigenous health workers. Efforts became more intense in relation to birth control in 1979. The one child family policy was promoted through extra benefits given to those that had only one child. Normal benefits were given for two children and for three there was a total loss of benefits. Family planning and contraceptive means were freely available and in rural areas a responsibility of the barefoot doctors.

Some would say the impact of health policy in China is impossible to evaluate because of an absence accurate statistics. Aggregation of health data beyond the local level was actively discouraged during the Cultural Revolution. It was reported that infant mortality in China's cities was reputed to have fallen from 120 per 1000 in 1949 to 12 per 1000 in 1981 and in rural areas from 200 per 1000 to between 20 and 30 per 1000 in 1981. Life expectancy was estimated at 69.6 for females and 67 for males in 1981 (Sidel & Sidel 1982, p. 91). While there remain doubts about the accuracy of some of the statistics, the evidence clearly points to a remarkable achievement in a short timespan. It has given hope to other countries, particularly in the third world, where such a model of modernisation offered more hope and was more relevant to poor largely rural third world nations. The World Bank World Development Report (World Bank 1981) summarised the international view on China's progress:

China's most remarkable achievement during the past three decades has been to make low-income groups far better off in terms of basic needs than their counterparts in most other poor countries. They all

Activities

- Discuss why a Western approach to health policy was unlikely to be effective in China.
- Do you feel it was right to use a lesser qualified worker as the principal health care provider?
- Discuss with your colleagues whether the Chinese model has anything to offer the Western world.

have work; their food supply is guaranteed through a mixture of state rationing and collective self-insurance; most of their children are not only at school but are also being comparatively well taught; and the great majority have access to basic health care and family planning services.

Discussion

When one considers the proportion of expenditure on health care of a selection of different countries it is clear that there is wide variation. The end result or judgement made regarding value for money or unit of health care, per dollar, is difficult to estimate. As one has seen from the brief outline of the countries considered, health care is not homogeneous. For example Germany and the USA are richer countries per capita than the United Kingdom. Using purchasing power parities, the index of GDP per capita in 1983 was: United States = 100; Germany = 82 and United Kingdom = 71 (Culyer 1990). This implies that the USA was on average 40% richer and Germany 15% richer than the United Kingdom. On face value if there was homogeneity in health care, both Germany and the USA would have more health service inputs than the United Kingdom. In practice, however, in 1983, while the United States had 60% more doctors per capita, they had 27% fewer hospital beds and 30% fewer nurses. Germany had 40% more beds than the United Kingdom but an incredible 85% more physicians than the United Kingdom and 59% fewer nurses (OECD 1988). Then when one considers a country such as China, which is very poor in comparisons of per capita income, there have been remarkable inroads made in relation to the health experience of its 1 billion citizens. It is clear from this that simply to look at the aggregated picture of expenditure only tells part of the story in relation to outcomes of health policy. The type of health policy pursued varies greatly from country to country. Why this should be so is not only to do with which approach is the best way of achieving a good outcome in terms of health experience of the population. There are other factors at work, such as the way professionals are paid and the

political influence they hold over the way the system is organised. In addition the way in which the system is administered and financed can be wasteful of the resources at its disposal. For example the US system of health insurance is costly and inefficient to run compared to the system of countries such as the United Kingdom that rely principally on taxation.

The future within most post-industrial nations is one where health policy is increasingly going to be dominated by the issue of priority setting and, ultimately, rationing of health care. Coast et al (1996) define rationing as the failure to provide all beneficial care to all people. By this definition it is already in evidence, with implicit and unacknowledged rationing occurring in all health systems (Regan 1988). It is generally accepted that rationing is necessary in the developed world and the debate is now more centred on the extent to which this is necessary. Knowledge about the effectiveness of different approaches, although poor, is improving. It is essential in all countries that new technology should not be introduced without proper evaluation, to prevent a demand being created for an expensive and possibly ineffective treatment. Few governments, if any, have taken responsibility for this as it proves rather unpopular (Abel-Smith 1994, p. 208). It is clear, particularly in most post-industrial economies, that health policy has been dominated by a biological and medical paradigm, principally how to provide the diagnosis and treatment of ill-health. This is increasingly being challenged by a socio-ecological paradigm which aims at prevention, health promotion and protection from the causes of ill-health. Another major change of emphasis is the holistic approach to the care of individuals, which challenges the dominance of professionals and their way of thinking (Abelin et al 1987). Ultimately it is the combination of both models that offers the greatest potential benefits in the future. However, as we have already seen in the United Kingdom, it can be difficult to redirect resources to promotion and prevention at the apparent expense of adopting the latest medical innovation in treatment of disease.

REFERENCES

Abel-Smith B 1994 An introduction to health: policy, planning and financing. Longman, New York

Abelin T, Brzezibski Z, Carstairs V (eds) 1987 Measurement in health promotion and protection. World Health Organization Regional Publications No. 22. WHO, Copenhagen

Bjorkman J 1991 Grains among the chaff – rhetoric and reality in comparative health policy. In: Altenstetter C, Haywood S (eds) Comparative health policy and the New Right: from rhetoric to reality. Macmillan, Basingstoke

Brannigan M 1995 Oregon's experiment. In: Seedhouse D (ed) Reforming health care: the philosophy and practice of international health reform, pp. 27–52. Wiley, New York

Coast J, Donavan J, Frankel S (eds) 1996 Priority setting: the health care debate. Wiley, Chichester

Culyer A J 1990 Cost containment in Europe. In: OECD Health care systems in transition. The search for efficiency, pp. 29–40. OECD, Paris

Feldstein P 1992 The changing structure of the health care delivery system in the United States. In: Rosenthal M, Frenkel M (eds) Health care systems and their patients: an international perspective. Westview Press, Oxford

Hackler C 1995 Health care reform in the United States. In: Seedhouse D (ed) Reforming health care: the philosophy and practice of international health reform, pp. 15–26. Wiley, New York

Ham C, Robinson R, Benjeval M 1990 Health check: health care reforms in an international context. King's Fund Institute, London

Inglehart J 1991 Germany's health care system. New England Journal of Medicine 324(7):503–508

Josefson D 1997 End to state regulation of health care costs in New York. British Medical Journal 314:168

Lindgren B 1990 Health care systems in transition. The Swedish health care system, pp. 74–79. OECD, Paris

Manning W, Newhouse J, Keeler E, Leibowitz A, Marquis M 1987 Health insurance and the demand for medical care: evidence from a randomized experiment. American Economic Review 77(3):251–277

Meyer J 1990 Health care systems in transition. The search for efficiency, pp. 115–118. OECD, Paris

Organization for Economic Cooperation and Development 1992 US health care at the cross-roads. OECD, Paris

Organization for Economic Cooperation and Development 1989 Health data file. OECD, Paris

Organization for Economic Cooperation and Development 1988: Measuring health care. Draft Report. MAS/WP1(88). OECD, Paris

Regan M 1988 Health care rationing. What does it mean? New England Journal of Medicine 319(17):1149–1151

Rosenthal M 1992 Modernization and health care in the People's Republic of China: the period of transition, pp. 293–315. In: Rosenthal M, Frenkel M (eds) Health care systems and their patients: an international perspective. Westview, Oxford

Rublee D A 1992 International health expenditure trends: the United States compared to other market oriented countries. In: Rosenthal M, Frenkel M (eds) Health care systems and their patients: an international perspective. Westview Press

Saltman R 1991 Nordic health policy in the 1980s. In: Altenstetter C, Haywood S (eds) Comparative health policy and the New Right: from rhetoric to reality, pp. 111–128. Macmillan, Basingstoke

Saltman R 1988 Health Care in Sweden. In: Saltman R B (ed) The international handbook of health care systems. Greenwood Press, London

Saltman R, von Otter C 1990 Planned markets and public competition: a framework for strategic reform in health systems. Cited in Altenstetter C, Haywood S (eds) Comparative health policy and the new right: from rhetoric to reality, p. 111. Macmillan, Basingstoke

Schubert-Lehnhardt V 1995 Who should be responsible for a nation's health? In: Seedhouse D (ed) The philosophy and practice of international health reform, pp. 167–170. Wiley, Chichester

Schulenburg J, Matthias G 1992 The German health care system: concurrent solidarity, freedom of choice, and cost control. In: Rosenthal M, Frenkel M (eds) Health care systems and their patients: an international perspective. Westview Press, Oxford

Sidel R, Sidel V 1982 The health of China. Beacon Press

Sidel V 1972 The barefoot doctors of the People's Republic of China. New England Journal of Medicine 286:1292–1299

Sonnefield S, Waldo D, Lemieux J, McKuisk D 1991 Projections of national health expenditures through the year 2000. Health Care Financing 13(1):1–27

Webber D 1991 Health policy and the Christian–Liberal coalition in West Germany: the conflicts over health insurance reform, 1987–88. In: Altenstetter C, Haywood S (eds) Comparative health policy and the New Right: from rhetoric to reality. Macmillan, Basingstoke

Wennstrom G 1992 New ideological winds are blowing in the Swedish health care system. In: Rosenthal M, Frenkel M (eds) Health care systems and their patients: an international perspective. Westview Press, Oxford

WHO 1981 Regional strategy for health for all. WHO, Copenhagen

Woolhander S, Himmelstein D 1991 The deteriorating administration efficiency of the United States health care system. New England Journal of Medicine 324(18):1253–1258

World Bank 1981 World development report. Oxford University Press, New York

Future trends

Julie S. Taylor   Fred Sutton   Kevin Gormley

At the end of this chapter the student will be able to:

- **discuss the evolutionary process of policy formulation**
- **consider indicators for future trends in health and social services**
- **discuss the potential of new services emerging as needs continue to change**

Introduction

Previous chapters have considered the implications of social policies on health and social care by examining some of the key features that have led to the environment in which health and social care is provided. This chapter will draw from the evidence provided by the past in an attempt to explore how some health and social services will unfold and new services emerge as we move into the next millenium and beyond.

When considering social policy in the future tense, there is a need to examine what needs to be done, what changes are needed, should the government take responsibility (Box 13.1)

Box 13.1 The role of the state

The four primary roles of the state (Webb 1985) are:

- strategic policy making
- financing the meeting of need
- service production
- safeguarding rights

---

and is this the only way of meeting this need? According to Webb (1985), United Kingdom social policy contains three core elements:

- An overall commitment to collective action to prevent, reduce or meet social needs, combined with public accountability in meeting them.
- An acceptance of a mixed economy of welfare involving state, voluntary, informal caring organisations.
- A clear explanation of public services, needs and expenditures.

From the beginning of their term in office, the present government expressed a continued commitment to the principles of the NHS. However, in their pre-election manifesto the Labour Party was equally clear in a further objective – the removal of health care as a contentious political issue. In doing so the government argues that it will permit progress to be made regarding the restructuring of services without having to worry about forthcoming elections or the latest opinion polls. Whether the government is able to achieve this or not will depend on major pressure groups, the support of trade unions and the attitude of opposition parties. The government also expressed a desire to continue with some health policies that were begun by the previous government, especially in areas such as primary health care, community care and increasing the use of information technology to ensure efficiency (Department of Health 1996a, b, c, d, e).

 Activity

Given the fact that there was a Conservative government for 18 years from 1979, list five things that you think would have been different in social policy had there been a different government.

POLITICAL PARTIES

The similarities between the main political parties are as important as their differences (George & Miller 1994). Both agree on low taxation,

although how low is debatable. Private ownership is seen as the most valued form of tenure by both parties, although they tend to disagree on the social housing sector and on the detail and extent of benefit schemes. All parties are agreed that the state has a role to play in universal and free schooling, but not on how this is administered (George & Miller 1994). Clearly, what constitutes an affordable welfare state is where the parties diverge.

With a Labour government, the NHS reforms of the last 18 years are likely to be modified. The New Right championed markets as an ideal way for individuals to participate by offering market choices, leading to decentralisation (Hill & Bramley 1986). This government, however, have promised to review GP fundholding, NHS trusts and the level of area health authority control. An interesting feature in regard to the creation of GP fundholders was the notion that patients and clients would have a much greater say about health care provision. One of the features of this was a move towards complementary health care, and indeed some practices began to employ counsellors and even aromatherapists and so on. Despite a demand for alternatives to traditional and mainstream therapies, they have not become as commonplace in health centres and hospitals as first envisaged.

HEALTH ECONOMICS

Since 1979 there has been a shift in emphasis in government policy. Before that year the main economic goal was the maintenance of full employment. Since then the government has committed itself to establishing a privately owned economy, pursuing higher rates of growth, with a general bearing down on inflation. The Labour Party has traditionally been a campaigner for full employment, but it too has recently changed its stance. There is, now, consent on both sides for pursuing policies for low income tax, with any increase in spending coming from the restructuring of public services, rather than an increase in funding.

If these policies continue, as seems likely, then the welfare state will become less affordable, and consequently degenerate. At times of economic stagnation or decline the demands on the welfare state increase, alongside calls for public spending to be curbed. The Conservatives tried to increase efficiency in services alongside measures to reduce demand, with a belief that market incentives will encourage economic growth. The economic growth that has occurred has not been sufficient to take up the reduction in government revenue.

With a reduction in direct taxation there has been an increase in indirect taxation, with the selling off of publicly owned utilities, but there has still been a shortfall in revenue and public spending. In order to balance out the welfare state, they will therefore either have to raise money elsewhere or slim down social services even more (George 1991).

One of the paradoxes of the NHS is that its successes can lead to its downfall. The introduction of new and more expensive technologies leads to a demand for these treatments through their very existence. Along with this improved health care, life expectancy has increased. Accordingly demand for health care has increased due to the ageing population. This increase in life expectancy has other implications for public spending. There is an increased demand for public services such as residential care and pensions. Coupled with this is the fact that people over retiring age are no longer contributing as much through income tax.

Most commentators, however, put forward new proposals which reduce expenditure and services rather than increase them. The present view seems to be that public expenditure is a drain on the nation's economic resources. It is extremely unlikely that revenues will be increased to meet the demand of extra spending. Both of the main political parties agree that increased taxation is undesirable. If there is to be no increase of taxation rates, coupled with the less than outstanding record of economic growth, then there will have to be a major restructuring of the welfare state.

Measures have been introduced to increase efficiency in the social services. Opinions on their success tend to depend on the political view-

point. The question that arises is, how far can you go down the road to increasing efficiency? The first move to greater efficiency tends to bring more gains than successive moves and there will come a point when moves to greater efficiency will have little effect on total public expenditure. If public expenditure is to be reduced, then there will have to be a reduction in public expenditure through reductions in social services. The main problem with this is that countries which neglect their social services neglect at the same time their future economic prosperity and their social cohesion and stability.

Activity

Organise a debate to identify the key ideological differences towards health care between the major political parties in Britain.

SOCIAL AND CLASS PROBLEMS

Earlier chapters have highlighted how social class and economic status have a direct influence on health. The 1997 annual report from the Office of National Statistics (Health Inequalities Decennial Supplement) shows that people at the lower end of the social scale have shorter lives and greater risks of ill-health and disability. From this report it would appear that progress in the last 2 decades has not been particularly good – the Black Report, published in the late 1970s, revealed similar findings. This was verified by the Chief Medical Officer who commented that although in general the nation's health had continued to improve, inequalities between the social groups had persisted as a serious and almost certainly increasing problem. In a recent seminar organised by the NHS Executive, evidence was provided showing that poorer health among the black and Asian population, due to specific diseases, continues to exist in comparison to the remainder of the population.

The situation that exists at present is not new. Differences between social groups have increased consistently since the 1930s (Power & Fox 1991). The Registrar General's classification of social class has been criticised because it is an incomplete guide. In spite of this inadequacy, it remains one of the few available tools to distinguish one group from another (Graham 1986). The problem with this limitation of available information lies in the fact that researchers frequently draw incorrect inferences, particularly so when they correlate social class with socioeconomic status.

Class and socioeconomic status (SES) are not interchangeable concepts. Social class alone cannot act as a reliable indicator of socioeconomic circumstances (Benzeval et al 1995) for the following reasons:

- women cannot be analysed as a single group because they often do not have an occupational label
- the SES of older people may bear little resemblance to their socioeconomic circumstances as determined by their previous occupation
- the occupations of minority ethnic groups is often recorded as higher than their actual lifestyle (for example they may own their business, but this may have to support a wide family structure)
- differences exist even within classes (for example GPs are classified the same irrespective of whether or not they are currently working)
- official statistics only provide children with a social class if the father is present (derived from Benzeval et al 1995, Graham 1986; Spencer 1993)

When alternative measures are used to collate an index of poverty, poorer districts have been shown to have higher incidences of mortality and morbidity rates than more wealthy areas (Reading 1993). A number of surveys have documented the role of poverty and family disadvantage on the rates of child abuse (Gil 1970, Wolfe & McGee 1991). Gibbons and colleagues (1990) used an Index of Social Disadvantage that included large family size, overcrowding, basic amenities and wage earning. The results from this survey revealed clear links between disadvantage and parenting problems. There are also significant differences in the material circumstances of families referred to social services for child care problems (Gibbons et al 1990). Graham (1993) uses the term hardship rather than poverty but nevertheless draws similar conclusions. In reviewing hardship and health in women's lives, she points out that seven out of ten children living with lone mothers receive less than 50% of the average wage. 'Economic disadvantage marks the pathways that women follow into lone motherhood' (p. 43). Of 1.1 million families claiming income support, only 33% contain a man (Graham 1993).

Activities

- Carry out a review of the literature of identify how social class and status continue to affect the level of health and well-being in Britain, and share your findings with your friends and teacher.
- Discuss ways that these issues could be addressed in a fair and equitable way.

UNEMPLOYMENT

In 1992, 33% of men without qualifications were unemployed, a rise of 23% since 1977. In the same year, only 10% of men who held degrees were unemployed, constituting a rise of only 6% (Benzeval et al 1995). Unemployment, in terms of lost revenue and benefits paid, costs the state at least £8000 per person every year. Most policy changes for the future, particularly in regard to reducing high levels of long term unemployment, will require extra resources, which will mean a balancing act between what is perceived as a necessary need and what is affordable. This juggling act will probably end in a pragmatic compromise working against those most in need. In Britain every single area of welfare provision has seen massive organisational change over the last few years, so much so that according to Williams (1992), we are now a country characterised by:

- fragmentation
- change and uncertainty
- contradiction.

The Minister of State at the Department of Social Security claims that the modern welfare state is one of a damaging dependency culture (Smith & Woods 1997). At the moment the benefits system interacts with the job market to discourage people taking up jobs, and we are all familiar with stories of people who will be worse off if they took a job. Individuals want to work, but low wages coupled with the loss of benefit means that, in reality, they are better off if they remain at home.

The notion that this vicious circle could be addressed by removing the poverty and employment traps whilst providing greater incentives and pressure to take up jobs is sound policy, but it is not new (Smith & Woods 1997). These authors highlight some of the lessons from Australia, which tightened its social security rules, introducing much more rigorous retraining requirements. Lone parents were offered jobs, education and training (JET) and child care became a priority. Despite the initial high outlay of such a scheme, by 1994 this strategy was recovering 90% of its costs.

Clearly education policy then has an indirect impact on health and it is exciting that this is one of the priority areas for attention with the new government. Unfortunately, in the real world of finite resources it is predicted that if current policies continue, the affordable welfare state will decline into a residual welfare state through inadequate funding more than through deliberate policy (George & Miller 1994). George & Miller (1994) contend that although in principle we cannot argue against increased efficiency, we can question the limits to which it is possible and the extent to which improvements in public services have been achieved only at the cost of living standards of the very people who work in these areas. 'There is a strong democratic case for giving the public the choice between a residual welfare state at a higher tax cost before

the former wins out by default on the assumption that it is the only way of squaring the welfare circle' (George & Miller 1994, p. 225).

FUNDING

The health service at the moment is gripped by a managerialist system that shows little evidence of being cost-effective, of helping patients, of efficiency, and certainly not of partnership. In fact, an enormous 11.6% of the NHS budget is currently spent on management (Numas 1997). The main evidence of any partnership has been in the emergence of 'New Social Welfare Movements' (Williams 1992), groups that were formed because of common unifying concerns for specific needs (for example HIV positive, survivors, disabled, carers and so forth).

Ham (1992) points out that countries which rely on tax or social insurance are generally more effective than those that rely on private insurance. In the USA there are 30 million people without medical insurance and many more are under-insured. He contrasts this with Sweden and Canada, where expenditure has stabilised. Holland and Germany provide good examples of inequality between people paying different sums of money for what amounts to the same care. This is unlikely to be seen as equitable in Britain though, and as Ham points out, social insurance is a middle way between taxed finance and private finance. This is an earmarked tax on a narrower tax base where individuals can see what happens to their contributions. In a proposed stakeholder society, this is a viable consideration (see also Box 13.2).

INDIVIDUAL RESPONSIBILITY

Within holistic health care systems concepts such as 'holism' and 'self-care' are often mentioned as desirable goals to be achieved. As long as these are objectives within an individual context they are worthy sentiments. On the other hand, it could be argued that 'self-care' within a framework of social policy smacks of personal responsibility again and is not always useful. However, it does offer some possibilities for the future and

Box 13.2 Labour health policy (derived from Ham 1992, Kenny 1997, Numas 1997)

Health policy under a Labour government:

- Labour will increase NHS funding
- Health authorities will be more democratic
- GP fundholding will disappear, replaced by locality commissioning
- There will be a new Mental Health Act with more emphasis on care in the community
- Integrated services that will involve housing, employment, leisure, transport and education
- District health authorities and FHSAs will be merged to allow comprehensive care planning at a local level
- A Health Technology Commission will be set up to provide early warning and promote cost-effective technologies
- Patients will actually come first
- There will be a broader programme of action to improve health which will involve increased health promotion and prevention
- A Minister of State for Community Care will be appointed
- Food scares are to be addressed with a new Food Standards Agency

those who did not and we are already aware that those on lower incomes have poorer health (Benzeval et al 1995). The basic state pension will remain, but the promised first priorities are to challenge assistance to those poorest pensioners and to help 1 million lone parents on income support to return to work by helping with child care and training opportunities (Grice & Smith 1997).

Activities

In groups, discuss the following three questions posed by Webb (1985, p. 290) and provide a short summary of your conclusions:

- What should be the future of statutory and non-statutory ways of meeting social needs and of resolving social problems?
- What ways of meeting social need are likely in practice to be adopted?

What are the likely implications of different ways of meeting need for social structure and political stability?

is central to the proposals of the Commission on Social Justice (1994), who suggest the following in addressing policy needs of the future:

- programmes to tackle unemployment
- a comprehensive re-employment service
- help for lone parents with child care
- intermediate labour markets (a sort of half-way house to the formal labour market in areas of high deprivation.

The Commission on Social Justice contends that current investment is insufficient, inflexible and irrelevant and that by encouraging lifelong saving Britain will be providing for its future. The prime minister has promised to shake up the £90 billion per annum welfare system with plans for a 'stakeholders welfare', where people will have a greater control over their contributions and the way they can draw on them. National Insurance contributions will be expanded, using half to fund the NHS and the other half going towards long term care for elderly. In 1989 individuals with occupational pensions had incomes over 50% higher than

PARTNERSHIP IN PAYING FOR SOCIAL SERVICES

While the government remains committed to a free at point of use health service, the same sentiments do not apply to social care services, particularly those that are provided for older people. This includes residential and domiciliary or home support services. In a policy document (Department of Health 1997), the government has stated that it will continue to keep the present funding system under review and that it agrees with the view of the Select Committee on Health (House of Commons 1996) that demographic and other pressures do not call for radical change in the medium term. This document goes on to state that the existing system can be improved on and proposes a number of ideas that would promote a greater public awareness of the costs people may face should they become dependent. The Consultation Paper 'A new partnership for care in old age' (Department of Health 1997) accepted the main conclusions of the earlier Consultation Paper,

'A new partnership for care' (Department of Health 1996). These include a commitment to: re-emphasise the importance of savings, through pensions and other means; regulate the selling and marketing of long term care insurance under the Financial Services Act; and to allow people to top up the residential care arranged by their local authority from resources disregarded by the means test. The desired effect of the partnership scheme will be twofold. First, it will balance the costs of providing social care services for older people, irrespective of whether they are living at home or in nursing or residential accommodation. Second, the partnership scheme will commit the government to contributing to the cost of care aside from the amount of money that the older person has accumulated.

According to the government (Department of Health 1997), people who have made provision to meet their care costs through insurance will now be able to protect more of their assets even if they receive means-tested public support for their residential care costs. At the same time the government remains committed to ensuring that people who genuinely cannot make provision for themselves are cared for properly. On this point the government aims to ensure that social care services, whether publicly or privately provided, and the health care services which complement them are of a high quality. Its plans for doing so are clearly set out in the recent White Papers on the health service, *The NHS: a service with ambitions* and *Primary health care* (Department of Health 1996a, b).

REGIONAL CONTROL

It has been proposed that the future for social policy may best be addressed by looking at some of the possibilities afforded by local diversity through devolution of some services currently managed centrally. Tuck (1995) argues that central government needs to free up the capital receipts held by local authorities as a consequence of council house sales and allow a major programme of house building and renovation. Accommodation for homeless or disadvantaged families could then be provided by proper

investment in social amenities and family support services.

Social agencies must be allowed to meet their obligations to children, families and communities under the Children Act. 'Simply expecting local authorities to direct existing, fully stretched resources away from child protection services as apparently advocated by the Department of Health is not in itself an adequate strategy' (Tuck 1995, p. 370). Interagency work is clearly a necessity but, as Tuck points out, at the moment this generally tends to be more on an individual case basis rather than working together as whole services in any meaningful way. It is clear that, within the NHS, it is 'no longer from Cradle to Grave, but from Pillar to Post' (Williams 1992, p. 202). The most important development in terms of regional responsibility will without doubt be an increasing focus on primary health care. The Primary Health Care Act emphasises the need for initiatives that address issues including collaboration, tackling health inequality and health action zones to deal with locally identified hot spots of ill-health.

Activities

- Discuss the advantages and disadvantages in delegating responsibility for health and social care services to regions.
- Contact your local council and health authority or even your member of parliament to find out their views on this subject.

THE WORLD HEALTH ORGANIZATION

In 1978, the World Health Organization and the United Nations Children's Fund jointly sponsored a world conference at Alma-Ata (then in the USSR). At this conference an initiative entitled Health for All by the Year 2000 was launched. It was designed to refocus international concepts for health, and health care provision, towards an agreed policy of community health promotion. Representatives of 134 nations, Britain included, affirmed the concept of health for all and issued the following declaration: 'by the year 2000 all the people of the world will have attained a level of health that will permit them to lead a socially and economically productive life' (WHO 1978). This, in turn, led to the launch of the World Health Organization's global strategy of Health for All by the Year 2000 (WHO 1981), which called for 'all people in all countries to have, at least, such a level of health that they ... may participate actively in the social life of the community in which they live'. In 1985, the WHO's European region published its own objectives for health for all (WHO 1985) (Box 13.3). It contained 38 European targets which translated into local programmes and confirmed a commitment to the global health for all strategy (Ashton 1992, Gormley 1995).

HEALTH PROMOTION

From its beginnings the National Health Service was supposed to provide a clear strategy reflecting health promotion and treatment of ill-health. However, in terms of allocating equal resources for both areas it is only in recent times that the government has began to focus on health

---

promotion issues. A number of documents identify the need to stimulate discussion regarding the potential for increasing the scope of modern preventive medicine within much wider parameters than the previous post-war boundaries, including: *Prevention and health: everybody's business* (DHSS 1976), *Priorities for health and personal social services in England* (DHSS 1976), *The way forward* (DHSS 1977), and the Acheson Report (DHSS 1988).

In line with these reports and other developments in primary health care, it became clear that the government had a much broader plan for the nature and function of the NHS. The government published a Green Paper, *The Health of the Nation* (Cm 1523 1991), which provided an outline for the future focus of health promotion. The following year the government published its final plan in the White Paper (DoH Cm 1986, 1992). This clarified the government's intention to address these health problems. The key change was an ideological shift towards policies supporting the Health for All strategy and an emphasis on addressing many of the structural and environmental influences on health (buildings, cars, recreational facilities, etc.). The White Paper was designed to refocus the service as a health service rather than simply a reactive ill-health service.

Box 13.3 European *Health for All* targets (adapted from Gormley 1995)

- Governments agreed to pursue policies that would both promote health and prevent illness
- Participating nations should work towards developing supportive environments for health which obliged nations not to pursue economic growth without first considering the ultimate health effects on its citizens in terms of the physical and social environment
- Consensus between the representative nations that health promoting services should be provided, equally and equitably. The WHO specifically targeted: women, children, ethnic minorities and the elderly
- The strategy also recommended the need for inter-sectorial action to encourage an integrated strategy for the promotion of health: water services, public transport services, health and safety, food hygiene and health organisations
- A commitment towards primary health care services (community health and social services) to encourage individual and community empowerment in health care decision making

---

Activities

- Discuss with your colleagues how the World Health Organization has affected the philosophy of the NHS.
- Discuss how you feel about these changes.

PRIMARY HEALTH CARE

Ewles & Simnett (1992) suggest that three definitions of health activity apply to the work of health care professionals. They are primary, secondary and tertiary care. Primary health care focuses on promoting a healthy lifestyle, secondary health care deals with existing ill-health and tertiary health care on optimising independence within the confines of existing disability. Primary health care has also been described as the continued health and social welfare offered appropriately to needful individuals living in private households (Rayner 1992, Jeffries 1995).

According to the figures contained in the government sponsored consultative document, *Primary care: the future* (NHSE 1996), the total spending on primary care (including community health services) is around £12.45 billion. This represents over 36% of total NHS spending. The document (NHSE 1996) went on to propose that primary health care staff should aim to improve partnership and foster an ethos towards community development. The document identified important development areas towards achieving this strategy. First, it aimed to ensure a fairer national distribution of primary care services. Second, it recommended a balance between the resources given to primary and secondary care. Third, it aspired to ensure greater flexibility in the use of local resources. Finally, the White Paper (Department of Health 1996) highlights a need to strengthen opportunities for encouraging personal growth and development for all primary health care staff particularly in areas such as information technology.

In 1996, the government also launched a period of consultation to look at the future direction for primary health care to create a renewed dynamic towards its further development (Department of Health 1996a). A number of complementary documents were published (NHSE 1996, Dept of Health 1996b, c, d). These publications preceded the release of a final White Paper, *Primary care: delivering the future* (Department of Health 1996). The White Paper, *The NHS: a service with ambitions* (Department of Health 1996) sets out the government's twin objectives for the NHS. First, it aims to have an 'integrated health service that meets the health needs of individual patients'. Second, it proposes that the NHS should balance the desire to provide care at home with the need to provide care that is safe. It goes on to describe the pivotal role of primary care as: skilled advice; treatment; health promotion and care in partnership with other professionals and agencies.

In the foreword to the White Paper (Department of Health 1996a), the minister for health proposed that the key demand made by professional staff during the consultation period was a call for partnership and community development to create a seamless service. This has been a constant objective since the launch of the Griffith Report in 1988 (DHSS 1988) and was reiterated in recent publications (Department of Health 1996a, b, c, d). The White Paper (Department of Health 1996a) specifically calls for improved collaboration between agencies at a strategic level and an individual level in order to meet the complex needs of older people (Para 2.22). According to the government, the White Paper (Department of Health 1996) reflects a demand for flexibility and allows for the tailoring of services to meet the needs of the public and professionals working in primary care.

In the government White Paper on primary health care (Department of Health 1996) a fairer distribution of resources across the country is promised, with a balance of resources between primary and secondary care. Underlying this is the belief that investing in primary care could help secondary care work more effectively (Secretary of State for Health 1996) (see also Box 13.4). Partnership between various agencies, in particular health and social services, is seen as of primary importance. Although there is some recognition that resources in the past have not always been fairly distributed, tangible evidence of a strategy to really get to grips with

---

Box 13.4 Proposals for the future

The former Secretary of State for Health (1996) outlined the following proposals that were aimed at addressing the principles of good primary care for the future. It was promised that:

- An extra £65 million will be put aside in cash limited funds
- £32 million in growth funds to be provided for hospital and community services to increase services between primary and secondary care
- Local health authorities will each spend £3000 on patient education campaigns in 1997/1998, working alongside the voluntary sector

health divisions has not yet been forthcoming. Within this climate it would be reasonable to suggest that new ideas of partnership, collaboration, fairness, public participation and reduced bureaucracy will perhaps supplant as ideals competitive tendering, the internal market and so on, terms that have been so fashionable since the Griffith period.

Activity

Discuss with your teacher the factors that have directed consecutive governments to focus on policies that focus on primary health care.

Conclusion

Webb (1985) points out that the basic options for the future are comparatively few, although there are complex variants and interactions between them. These are summarised thus:

- a radical shift away from or towards more state involvement
- effect more modest and reformative changes in the existing balance between statutory and non-statutory involvement
- adopt new philosophies, objectives, operational goals and approaches to management.

So what will the future look like? It would be wonderful to paint a rosy picture of the year 2041, when I could be considering entering residential, 'hotel-type' accommodation paid for by my state pension that has plenty left every week to pay for my state of the art moon buggy/wheelchair. My grandchildren and great-grandchildren need never fear living in poverty, because the state has sorted out welfare provision to such an extent that the disadvantages faced by certain sectors of society have been abolished.

In all probability the same level of ill-health, with its linkage with class and socioeconomic differences will continue. However, it is not all doom and gloom. Some believe the terminal

decline of the NHS has been exaggerated and the predicted health care rationing is avoidable (Flemming & Oppenheimer 1996). Small steps first – we may resolve key tensions in social policy by, for example, citizenship, the provision of a basic income which extends outside the labour market, or with low cost housing that is not dependent on assumptions of what constitutes a 'normal' family (Williams 1992). Most essentially though, we need to grasp the fact that the most significant causes of mortality and morbidity occur at the social level (Baggott 1994), and use this knowledge to effect real change in the areas where we work. Only by doing this can we have any impact on the wider policies that exist outside of our direct sphere of influence.

It would seem that the threshold of what constitutes 'normal' is socially and culturally defined (Department of Health 1995). We have lived through substantial cultural and social changes that only become apparent on historical reflection. Technological advances aside, cultural and sociological changes such as living together before marriage do not raise many eyebrows these days, and piercing parts of the body beyond the ear lobes is reasonably common. A few years from now there will be a whole ward of elderly women who have tattoos in interesting places and more men may be staying at home looking after the children. 'Eco-warriors' like Swampy have already appeared as celebrities on television game shows. Headline news about surrogate or gay parents will probably attract as much attention tomorrow as giving birth out of wedlock does today.

From the evidence it would appear that as services continue to expand away from institutional care, professionals in the field will become important players in policy development and implementation. Already health care professionals are expected to practice in different ways across a wide range of boundaries and institutional settings. At present health care professionals are not significantly influential in the higher political echelons. This does not mean, however, that things will not change. As Numas (1997) predicts in rather evocative terms, 'The voice of the silent majority, including nurses, patients and other NHS employees, will need to beome audible again and, more importantly, listened to by the decision-makers' (Numas 1997, p. 30). In order to achieve this, health care professionals must understand the complexities of the present within a wider context, which should enable us to be proactive deliverers of the very best health care in the future.

Activities

- Use a brainstorming session to generate a list of what you think you will see in terms of attitude change in the next 20 years.
- In pairs, use this list as the basis of discussion regarding your perceived changes in health policy for the new millennium.

REFERENCES

Ashton J 1992 Healthy cities project. Open University Press, Milton Keynes

Baggott R 1994 Health and health care in Britain. Macmillan, Basingstoke

Benzeval N, Judge K, Whitehead M 1995 Unfinished business. In: Benzeval N, Judge K, Whitehead N Tackling inequalities in health. An agenda for action; pp. 122–140. King's Fund, London

Commission on Social Justice 1994 Social justice: strategies for national renewal. The report of commission on social justice. Vintage, London

Department of Health 1995 Child protection. Messages from research. HMSO, London

NHSE 1996 Primary care: the future. HMSO, London

Department of Health 1996a Cmnd 3512, Primary care: delivering the future. HMSO, London

Department of Health 1996b The National Health Service: a service with ambitions. HMSO, London

Department of Health 1996c Patients not paper. HMSO, London

Department of Health 1996d Developing emergency services in the community. HMSO, London

Department of Health 1996e Assessing older people with dementia in the community: practice issues for social and health services. HMSO, London

Department of Health 1997a Health services for children and young people in the community: home and school. HMSO, London

Department of Health 1997b The health survey for England, 1995. HMSO, London

Flemming J, Oppenheimer P 1996 Are government spending and taxes too high (or too low)? National Institute Economic Review 157:57–77

George V, Miller S 1994 2000 and beyond. A residual or a citizen's welfare state? In: George V, Miller S Social policy towards 2000, pp. 215–239. Routledge, London

Gibbons J, Thorpe S, Wilkinson P 1990 Family support and prevention: studies in local areas. National Institute for Social Work/HMSO, London

Gil D G 1970 Violence against children: physical child abuse in the United States. Harvard University Press, Cambridge, MA

Gormley K 1995 Health promotion and education for self care. In: Basford L, Slevin O Theory and practice of nursing: an integrative approach to patient care. Campion Press, Edinburgh

Graham H 1986 Caring for the family. Health Education Council, London

Graham H 1993 Hardship and health in women's lives. Harvester Wheatsheaf, New York

Grice A & Smith D 1997 Blair launches crusade for welfare reform. The Sunday Times: 1, 4th May

Ham C 1992 Health policy in Britain. Macmillan, Basingstoke

Hill M, Bramley G 1986 Analysing social policy. Basil Blackwell, Oxford

Numas R 1997 New Labour, new NHS. Nursing Times 93(20):30–31

Power C, Fox J 1991 Health and class: the early years. Chapman and Hall, London

Reading R 1993 Geography as an indicator of social disadvantage. In: Waterston T Perspectives in social disadvantage and child health, pp. 27–30. Intercept Ltd, Newcastle-upon-Tyne

Secretary of State for Health 1996 Primary care: delivering the future. Department of Health, London

Smith D, Woods R 1997 How will they fare? The Sunday Times. London: 5.6, 11th May

Spencer N 1993 Social disadvantage and child health – a medical perspective. In: Waterston T Perspectives in social disadvantage and child health, pp. 9–15. Intercept Ltd, Newcastle-upon-Tyne

Tuck V 1995 Links between social deprivation and harm to children. A study of parenting in social disadvantage. Unpublished PhD thesis. Social Sciences, Psychology. University of Warwick, Coventry

Webb A 1985 Alternative futures for social policy and state welfare. In: Berthoud R Challenges to social policy, pp. 46–71. Gower, Aldershot

Williams F 1992 Somewhere over the rainbow: universality and diversity in social policy. In: Manning N, Page R Social policy review 4, pp. 200–219. Social Policy Association, London

Wolfe D A, McGee R 1991 Assessment of emotional status among maltreated children. In: Starr R, Wolfe D A The effects of child abuse and neglect. Issues and research, pp. 257–277. Guilford Press, New York

World Health Organization 1978a Constitution. In Basic Documents. WHO, Geneva

World Health Organization 1978b Alma-Ata. Primary Health Care. Health for All Series No. 1. WHO, Geneva

World Health Organization 1981 Global strategy for health for all by the year 2000. WHO, Geneva

World Health Organization 1985 Targets in support of the European strategy of health for all. WHO, Geneva

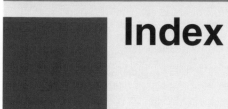

Index